Lean and Fit
A Doctor's Journey to Healthy Nutrition and Greater Wellness

JOSEPH E. SCHERGER, MD, MPH

DEDICATION

To my mentor physicians, William Davis, David Perlmutter,
Mark Hyman and my partner in practice
(and personal physician) Hessam Mahdavi,
all champions of Functional Medicine.

To Robert Atkins, Jeff Volek and Stephen Phinney for
advancing the science of low carbohydrate nutrition.

To Daniel Lieberman at Harvard for teaching us
about the human body.

ACKNOWLEDGMENT

To Helen Searing, my assistant at
Eisenhower Medical Center,
who worked diligently to make this book
come out so well.

To my son Adrian Scherger who inspires me to write
and helped with the cover and making this book
more appealing to readers.

LEAN AND FIT

CONTENTS

Appendices: 73-93

About the Author   95

PREFACE

A Doctor's Journey to Healthy Nutrition and Greater Wellness

Why do we keep poisoning ourselves? We do not know any better. Sure we think we do. It must be the sugary beverages, or the supersizing of french fries at fast food restaurants. Those are problems but they are not the big picture. The real cause of the poisoning that has made most of us overweight or obese, with a staggering burden of diseases, is a toxic food environment of high glycemic carbohydrates and inflammatory proteins. As the famed evolutionary biologist from Harvard, Daniel Lieberman, has written, cultural evolution has given us a diet and lifestyle that does not match our bodies, and we are in a state of disevolution.

I know this sounds extreme. Aren't bread and cookies and cupcakes and brownies and bagels and ice cream normal foods? No they are not. Look around. The majority of people are seriously overweight and more than 1 in 3 are obese. Diabetes, type 1 and 2, do not need to happen. The auto-immune diseases, from lupus to rheumatoid arthritis to hypothyroidism do not need to happen. Autism and multiple sclerosis and Parkinson's disease and Alzheimer's disease do not need to happen. Acne and rosacea do not need to happen. High blood pressure and high cholesterol do not need to happen. Acid reflux and irritable bowel syndrome do not need to happen. All are diseases of our malnutrition.

We evolved to eat the foods nature gives us – vegetables, fruits, nuts, seeds, fish and meat from animals fed on the land. We have never had such a variety and abundance of these foods available. Yet we have created foods that harm us such as breads and other flour based foods, and sweets. Hospitals continue to serve unhealthy food. We entice doctors and medical students to come to meetings by serving pizza or bagels. We reward our police and ambulance drivers by giving them doughnuts. We celebrate by having parties that serve cake. The inconvenient truth, as this book will describe, is that these pleasurable foods are hurting us in very serious ways.

The biology of human health is poorly understood. We know a lot about our organs and our organ systems, but what constitutes health is not well known and hence is argued at a basic level. We are sustained by what we eat yet what constitutes the right healthy diet is highly controversial and keeps changing. We have recently discovered a new "organ system", the human microbiome, and that may turn out to be the most important of all.

This book is about my health, a family doctor with a career long interest in preventive medicine as much as my interest in disease. As someone who has always strived to be healthy, at age 63, just two years ago, much of what I thought was healthy nutrition has changed. As I used new knowledge to change my nutrition, my health went from good to great.

I share this journey, and some of the articles I have written, in hopes that it will help you become healthier. Everyone's life is a journey and we make many choices along the way. Far better health and longevity with a greater healthspan are within our reach. We are designed to be lean and fit, yet there are powerful forces working against us, especially in the United States. But knowledge is power and hopefully you will find some of my journey useful as you navigate your way to better health.

Joseph E. Scherger, MD, MPH
October, 2015

JOSEPH E. SCHERGER, MD, MPH

PART 1: 63 YEARS OF MOSTLY GOOD HEALTH

I came from a family with a strong health orientation in the small town of Delphos, Ohio in the Northwestern part of the state that resembles the flat farmlands of the Midwest. My home town of 7000 people was surrounded by corn fields and wheat fields. My father was president of the local bank and spent much of his time lending money to farmers. Our family kept an eye out for health news and I was raised on a lot of whole wheat bread and cow's milk. My parents reverted to skim milk when the low fat products were promoted.

Both my parents lived into their early 90s, so I have good genes. My father suffered near the end of his life with Parkinson's disease and eventually the dementia that accompanies that dreadful neurodegenerative illness. He died a shadow of his former self. My mother suffered from gallbladder disease and died two years after my father mainly to join him in heaven.

Growing up my favorite food was bacon and I would always order 10 strips from an obliging mother who lived by the philosophy "feed them what they will eat". In high school I had two hot dogs almost every night before bed with a glass of milk. I was not a good athlete in the three team sports, football, basketball and baseball, but I stayed lean and fit riding a bicycle most everywhere and playing golf and tennis.

My big nuisance health problem was acne. It started like most teenagers at puberty but it did not want to go away as I became an adult. I was embarrassed often in medical school with big zits in my 20s. Finally in my 50s the pimples receded but I developed an adult form of acne, rosacea on and around my nose. In my early 60s I was applying an antibiotic gel on and around my nose twice a day until I discovered what was causing the problem, but that story is in the next part of this book.

I was healthier at 30 than I was at 20. At age 20 I was studying hard in college in order to get to medical school and I got very little exercise. I never become overweight in my 20s but I had limited muscle strength and by today's standards would be called a nerd. In my late 20s finishing my medical training in family medicine and public health, I joined the running craze that developed in the 1970s. I started my medical practice in the college town of Davis, California and my neighbor was a runner. He invited me to join him in the Runner's World 12 week training schedule to run a marathon. I was already running about 30 minutes on most days so I was ripe for this effort.

Our first race was the Bay to Breakers 8 mile run in San Francisco that was so much fun I was hooked. Our first marathon in 1979, me at age 29, was the President's Cup in San Francisco that was held only once because the police said no way they would block that much traffic again. We started on Treasure Island in San Francisco Bay and ran over the Bay Bridge to the Embarcadero. We ran by all the piers and through the Presidio and went back and forth over the Golden Gate Bridge. The 26.2 miles ended in Golden Gate Park. My neighbor was quite fast and made his goal of less than 3 hours to qualify for Boston. We ran three marathons together over three years and with his fast pace inspiration I finished them between 3:15 and 3:30, despite getting only water along the way and hitting the "wall" around 20 miles as the muscles ran out of carbohydrate energy. At age 30 I was lean and fit weighing 155 pounds at 5 feet 11 inches. I had a 32 inch waist. I felt like the statue of David.

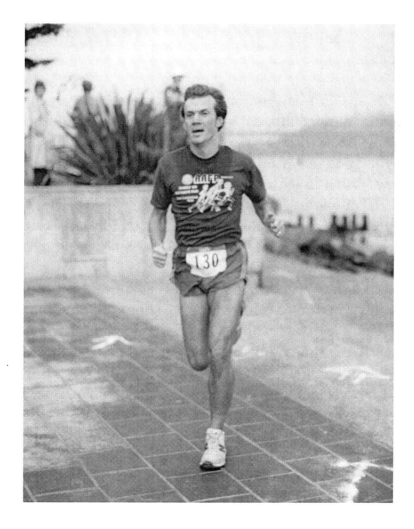

In 1982 my neighbor moved away and I became very busy with my medical practice. My running tapered off to the occasional 5k. By age 46 my weight was 192 pounds, my peak, and not good. My total cholesterol was 211 and my HDL (good cholesterol) was only 37.

Despite my parents' longevity, heart disease runs in our family and I was at risk. I faced the decision to go on a statin or lose the weight. One of my two sons inspired me to become a runner again and do marathons. That seemed the healthy choice. I also cut out some of the fat in my diet such as salad dressings and butter on bread, decisions I would not make today.

By age 63 I had run 30 marathons and had even started running ultramarathons at age 61 after reading the life altering book, *Born to Run* by Christopher McDougall. My weight came down to 180 on this plan and my cholesterol dropped to 175 with HDL cholesterol of 52. No statin for me and it shows how exercise and weight loss can lower total cholesterol and raise the HDL. Oddly my waistline was still 36 inches. At 180 pounds I was a heavy runner.

At age 57 I developed another health problem. I became mildly hypothyroid, a common autoimmune problem. I knew something was not quite right. I felt a little sluggish, my running became slower and it was hard to lose weight. Sure enough my TSH was above the normal range. That corrected with a modest dose of levothyroxine. Why had I developed this problem with no family history of hypothyroidism? I would find out why later.

I am also a medical writer and my first book is a collection of articles I have written over my 40-year career.

I share two of them here that reflect my focus on good health and the benefits of running that come from this period of my life.

Teaching a Healthy Lifestyle

Hippocrates
2000;14(1):7-8

The rules are simple. They have been known for a long time. They are more important than ever.

A century ago, living a healthy lifestyle might not have given much assurance for a long and healthy life. If you acquired a serious bacterial infection or appendicitis, chances were you would die. We have conquered many of the causes of premature death that plagued mankind prior to the twentieth century. Now, as we enter the twenty-first century, good health and a long life are more than ever a choice.

Sure, genetics, infections, accidents, or cancers may end life early for some, but lifestyle factors now loom as the leading cause of premature death. Promoting a healthy lifestyle must now become a principal focus for primary care physicians.

Despite the extravagant claims of supplement manufacturers, good health does not come in a bottle. A "fountain of youth" craze seems to come over the population periodically, a hope for simple external solutions to what is an internal issue. The 1890s were the decade of patent medicines, with a proliferation of nostrums promising good health. Curiously, we saw a similar public fascination with unproved medications in the 1990s as pharmacies all over the country devoted expanding amounts of square footage to nutritional supplements that promised various health benefits. Truth and common sense usually prevail, and I suspect this current preoccupation will pass. Perhaps then we will have a more receptive audience for our teaching of the timeless rules of healthful living. These rules are straightforward – we heard most of them first from our parents – but coming from a personal physician they can be a powerful prescription. I offer these 10 simple rules as a reminder to ourselves and as a message to share with our patients.

Don't Smoke

I hate to lead off with a negative recommendation, but tobacco use is the number one cause of premature death in this country. We should not lose sight of that lest we let our guard down. With tobacco use rising again among high school and college students we must redouble our efforts to combat this social menace. We need to work hard to prevent and eliminate smoking one patient at a time – in the exam room, in our schools, and in our communities. Be active in smoking prevention and learn strategies for teaching patients how to kick the habit.

Be Active

The evidence supporting the health benefits of physical activity and the consequences of inactivity are so compelling that this rule rises to number two. Many adults have become more physically active in the last two decades, contributing to the decline in heart disease. However, a growing number of young people are not physically active, and obesity among children is on the rise. Work at home and on the job is less physically demanding today, and conscious choices must be made to walk and get other forms of exercise. Recent research shows that all physical activity counts and its benefits are cumulative. As we make time for exercise in our own busy lives, we should regularly inquire about our patients' activity levels and instruct them about being active.

Eat Right

Note the dietary advice below reflects what I wrote, taught and practiced in 2000. Today I would encourage foods from natural sources such as vegetables, nuts, seeds and whole fruit. I would not restrict fat from these sources and I would specify fiber from these foods rather than from grains.

Just what this means seems more confusing than ever, as "protein diet" books dominate the best-seller lists and carbohydrates are considered either a blessing or curse, depending on the diet. The real problem today is that an excessive amount of food is readily available, even to low-income Americans. Eating out can rival the cost of eating at home and is often easier. Jumbo-sized fast-food meals are commonplace. Unhealthy fat abounds in such foods as french fries, potato chips, and salad dressings. Eating right means not consuming more energy than you burn and making wise choices. The food pyramid is a big improvement over the four food groups and teaching its use promotes a low-fat, high-fiber diet, the healthiest combination. Effective nutritional interventions with patients must be sensitive to personal preferences, which may be culturally based. Start with the patient's own food diary and be flexible. Promote healthy eating.

Be Happy

I am not suggesting a false sense of bliss, but having a positive outlook does have health benefits. My first "patient" in this regard was my freshman college roommate. To him, life was a joyless, uphill struggle. He grew up on Long Island, the son of an industrial assembly line worker. I am proud to say that now with persistent counseling from myself and others he is a remarkably healthy and optimistic school superintendent. Depression is now regarded as a leading cause of disability worldwide. Mental health is critically important to overall health. In any way we can, we should model and promote positivity.

Relax

In the complexity of modern life, it is easy to be "all wound up." Do any of us have idle time? The body and mind need to relax, and probably more often than just during sleep. The integrative medicine article reports on the benefits of meditation, or deep relation. As with exercise, we need to make time for this fundamentally healthy activity. Promote relaxation with patients.

Have Purpose

George Engel suggested a biopsychosocial model for medicine in the 1970s. The growing evidence regarding spirituality and health suggests a connection. Purpose, or having a higher meaning to your life than mere existence, seems to be important for overall health. Explore this dimension with patients. For patients who don't have a social group or are not involved in their communities, for example, promote greater involvement.

Be Safe

Accidents loom large as a preventable cause of death, especially among the young. Instruct patients to wear seat belts or bicycle helmets, use infant car seats, and drive safely. Components of home safety such as smoke detectors, safe appliances and electrical wiring, gun locks, and fences around pools may be lifesaving. Safety lectures may be the last thing on a busy practitioner's mind, but accidents are the fifth leading cause of death in the U.S. Any effort physicians can make to prevent accidents is effort well spent.

Sleep Well

We should be spending between one third and one quarter of our lives in sound sleep. Poor sleep habits are common and the health consequences are becoming known. Most fibromyalgia patients improve with better sleep. Drowsiness kills on highways. We train our children to sleep, sometimes a challenging task, but as adults we often fall into poor sleep habits and lack a "parent" to set us straight again. We will have more emphasis on sleep hygiene as evidence comes in regarding the health benefits of good sleep.

Counsel Safe Sex

Many of the serious and incurable infections of our time, such as HIV and hepatitis B and C, are transmitted sexually. Being careful and using protection in sex is a health imperative for anyone not in a long-term, monogamous relationship. Teaching adolescents and adults a healthy lifestyle must include this precaution.

Use Moderation

My mother, like many, counseled "Everything in moderation." She was right. Moderation is important in several health-related behaviors. Light-to-moderate alcohol consumption has demonstrated health benefits. Alcohol should be consumed safely, which generally means at home. Moderate exercise makes the most sense for many, especially the elderly. Eating moderately means saying no to super-sized fries and desserts. Moderation is a wise principle to live by.

Why Do I Run?

Hippocrates
2000;14(6):8

	1997	**2000**
Weight:	190 lb.	175 lb.
Total Cholesterol:	211 mg/dl	160 mg/dl
HDL Cholesterol:	37 mg/dl	51 mg/dl

Those are my vital statistics. What made the difference? Twenty miles a week and a reduction in dietary fat.

As I am about to turn 50, my health becomes a high priority. My first weight and lipid panel, two years ago, frightened me. I had always been lean and healthy. Too many restaurant dinners and too little time for physical activity were taking their toll. One of my sons challenged me to get back in shape and run a marathon with him. He reminded me that I'd run three when he was a child. That was just the push I needed.

I learned from *Galloway's Book on Running* to train for a marathon by running just 20 to 25 miles a week. Such a regimen accommodates my busy life and my biologic need, as a runner over 40, for 48 hours of recovery between longer runs. After just four months of training, my weight was down and my lipids much better. Since the first marathon I ran with my son, on Father's Day in 1998, I have run three, including the Boston Marathon in April. I'm running another in June. Today I feel better than I did when I turned 40.

I resumed running for the health benefits, but to keep myself motivated, I needed a concrete goal. A marathon to look forward to periodically serves that purpose.

The benefits of regular physical activity are well documented. Going from unfit to fit reduces all-cause mortality by as much as 44%. Besides reducing the risk of cardiovascular disease, regular physical activity reduces colon cancer risk, improves glucose control, increases insulin sensitivity, and lowers blood pressure. Recent studies in mice even suggest it may stimulate the growth of brain cells, thus reducing the risk of memory loss.

In the last five years, research has proven that even moderate physical activity helps. We should counsel our inactive patients to include more physical activity in their daily routines – walking more, taking the stairs, doing things by hand. Structured exercise is the second step, and we should advise patients that making time for it may be just as vital to their health as eating and sleeping.

The mental health benefits of exercise are as important as the physical effects. The same son who encouraged me to resume running two years later suffered a near-fatal auto accident on January 1, 2000. Running helped me deal with the stress of his tragedy and the hard work of helping him recover.

Being sedentary carries its own risks: It contributes substantially to the likelihood of coronary heart disease, Type 2 diabetes, and colon cancer – all potentially fatal. In 1992, the American Heart Association named physical inactivity as an independent risk factor for cardiovascular disease. Recent evidence shows that lack of cardiorespiratory fitness may be more of a health risk than obesity.

Promoting regular physical activity is a challenge worth taking on with all patients. We need to individualize our advice: patients will have their own ways of – and reasons for – being active. I do not entirely enjoy running marathons. They are painful, but the pain is quickly forgotten, I replaced by a sense of accomplishment. Sharing my marathon experiences with patients can help them find their own motivation for making exercise a part of their lives.

Breast cancer survivor Peggy Fleming calls exercise her "foundation of youth." The benefits have been known for centuries:

"Better to hunt in fields, for health unbought,
Than fee the doctor for a nauseous draught.
The wise, for curse, on exercise depend;
God never made his work for man to mend."
John Dryden

PART 2: DROP THE WHEAT AND LOSE THE WEIGHT

I am an avid "reader" of recorded books. There has been a book in my car continuously for the last 30 years. First it was Books on Tape and I went through many boxes. Then it became CDs. Now I use Audible.com, a subsidiary of Amazon and the books download into my iPad and are Bluetoothed into my car's sound system. I listen to all kinds of nonfiction where I think I can learn something. I am a history buff and learn a lot from good biographies of people I admire. I do enjoy the occasional novel. With Audible.com I get a "Daily Deal" in my morning email offering a book that day for less than $5. One day in September, 2013, at age 63, the Daily Deal was *Wheat Belly* by Dr. William Davis. I studied nutrition when getting my Masters in Public Health (MPH) at the University of Washington in 1978 and followed the latest nutrition recommendations carefully. I preached and practiced the low fat high fiber from whole grain diet. This book looked interesting.

Good books can change your life and *Wheat Belly* did just that. With great detail backed up by good scientific references, Dr. Davis described the two health problems caused by modern wheat. First is the heavy carbohydrate load and it became clear that the heavy intake of carbohydrates is the main problem behind the overweight and obesity epidemic. Carbohydrates drive hunger and when we ingest more of them we eat more. The epidemic of overweight and obesity coincided with the development of the low fat food industry. Low fat means more carbohydrates. Turns out Robert Atkins back in the 1970s was right after all and the American Heart Association and the American Diabetes Association got it wrong.

The second health problem with wheat is the inflammatory proteins. These proteins found in all grains appear to cause a wide range of health problems. The most famous of the inflammatory proteins is the gluten complex in wheat, barley and rye. Gluten is not a single protein but a complex of proteins mainly consisting of gliadin and gutenin. Gliadin is the most inflammatory. Celiac disease is an extreme form of gluten intolerance and those who suffer cannot ingest even trace amounts of wheat. However, it appears that we all may suffer from what is being called non-celiac gluten sensitivity.

I listened to this book not just once but twice and then ordered 15 hard copies. To be sure I learned everything I could from this book I read it in print form and gave the others out to friends and recommended it for patients.

I gave up all foods made with flour and changes began to happen quickly. I started losing weight without dieting almost like magic. What is amazing is that when you give up these high glycemic foods the hunger drive seems to disappear. After a breakfast I will describe later, I was not hungry by lunch time and would eat less. A smaller dinner of a good entrée and vegetables was totally satisfying. No more food cravings.

In addition, by going off gluten my rosacea went away! I learned from Chapter 12 of *Wheat Belly* that my acne for so many years and later rosacea were caused by the inflammatory effects of gluten. Gluten also set me up for the autoimmune problem of hypothyroidism. I will be on thyroid medication the rest of my life thanks to wheat.

As I made this rapid health transformation I was inspired to read more books. I followed *Wheat Belly* with *Grain Brain* by neurologist and nutritionist Dr. David Perlmutter. Perlmutter focuses on how elevated blood sugar from grains and sweets accelerates brain atrophy and increases the progression to dementia. From him I learned the importance of getting my fasting blood sugar to less than 90 and getting my HbA1c, a test for control of diabetes, to the lowest level possible. HbA1c is a measurement of the average blood sugar over 3 months by looking at how much sugar coats our red blood cells that live in our body for about 3 months. The lower blood sugar, the sharper our mind. In addition, the inflammatory protein complex gluten has a toxic effect on the brain and most likely causes neurodegenerative disease such as multiple sclerosis and Alzheimer's disease.

Health and longevity are not just about a great lipid panel and avoiding dementia, cancer looms as a cause of about one third of premature deaths. An academic nutritionist and cancer epidemiologist, Colin Campbell at Cornell, was frustrated that his more than 400 scientific papers contained vital health information but were not known to the public. He went public with his 2006 book, *The China Study*. What I read first was his 2013 book, *Whole: Rethinking the Science of Nutrition*. Campbell is a champion of a whole food plant based diet after finding the populations that lived all or mostly on vegetables lived healthier and longer lives, and had the lowest rates of cancer. Campbell is a hero of the vegan diet and even claims that following it carefully may help reverse some cancers. I wonder why all cancer centers do not promote a whole food plant based diet.

I wrote a collective book review of *Wheat Belly*, *Grain Brain* and *Whole* for the journal *Family Medicine* which is reprinted here:

Big Ideas in Nutrition: Three Books Worth Knowing

Book Review
Family Medicine
2014;46(9):726-727

Wheat Belly. William Davis, M.D. Rodale. 2011.

Grain Brain. David Perlmutter, M.D. Little, Brown and Co. 2013.

Whole: Rethinking the Science of Nutrition. T. Colin Campbell, PhD, Howard Jacobson, PhD. BenBella Books. 2013.

Let food by thy medicine and medicine be thy food.
Hippocrates

No disease that can be treated by diet should be treated by any other means.
Maimonides

Much has happened in food science since the recommended four food groups of the 1950s. With emerging evidence about heart disease caused by atherosclerosis and the role of cholesterol, low saturated fat diets were promoted. Unfortunately, many people replaced saturated fats with high glycemic carbohydrates and the overweight, obesity and type 2 diabetes epidemics took off in 1980. Robert Atkins first promoted a low carbohydrate diet in the 1972 book, *Dr. Atkin's Diet Revolution*. Food pyramids and many other diets followed.

Three recent books are reviewed here that may have a major impact in how we can use nutrition to combat the burden of disease. The lack of nutrition education in medicine is well known. Emerging information from nutrition science calls on medicine to heed the admonitions of Hippocrates and Maimonides.

William Davis is a preventive cardiologist in Milwaukee and in his practice promotes a wheat-free diet to lose weight and restore health. The book is well referenced and stays focused on two areas where wheat causes health problems. First he argues that modern engineered wheat with its 42 chromosomes is much different from the 14 chromosome einkorn wheat man began to eat 10,000 years ago and until the last century. Modern wheat is energy dense with the highly glycemic amylopectin A causing blood sugars to rise rapidly and remain high, even more so than many other sweets. The resulting rise in insulin levels causes the deposition of fat, especially central fat.

The second problem with modern wheat is the protein complex known as gluten. Gluten is actually a variety of proteins unique to wheat, barley and rye. Gliadins and glutenins are the two main types of gluten and we measure antibodies to these to test for gluten sensitivity. Inflammatory reactions to gluten are common and Davis argues that this is likely a basis for much auto-immune disease such as inflammatory arthritis and hypothyroidism. Direct inflammatory reactions to gluten may play a leading role in esophageal reflux, irritable bowel disease, acne and rosacea. In *Wheat Belly*, most chapters are focused on the impact of wheat on different organ systems. The evidence here is suggestive and the references are given, and much work needs to be done to nail down what is true.

In *Grain Brain*, David Perlmutter, a neurologist in Naples, FL with a graduate degree in nutrition, argues that wheat and other high glycemic sugars are the basis of much neurodegenerative diseases such as multiple sclerosis, Parkinson Disease and Alzheimer's dementia. He argues that the inflammatory nature of gluten and the toxicity of hyperglycemia damage the nervous system. The problem with this book compared with *Wheat Belly* is that it loses focus and Perlmutter lapses into a promotion of eating saturated fats *(he was right!)* and taking many supplements.

T. Colin Campbell is a highly respected nutrition scientist from Virginia Tech and then Cornell most famous for a large epidemiologic study in Asia called *The China Study* (BenBella Books, 2005). Campbell is well published in scientific journals but went public to get his information better known. He argues for a whole food plant based diet and that animal proteins correlate with many cancers. Casein, the protein in cow's milk, seems to be the worst especially correlating with breast and prostate cancer.

Campbell is a champion of many vegans and Bill Clinton has become an advocate. In *Whole,* Campbell and Jacobson reiterate the data from *The China Study* and argue why reductionist science alone cannot give the answers we need in nutrition. He uses the example of the synergy in an apple when eaten whole gives far more anti-oxidant activity than any of its known ingredients individually. His argument against taking supplements that confuse the body and lack the synergy of whole foods is especially powerful.

Taken together, these three books provide important information about nutrition. We are what we eat and medicine continues to lack sufficient education in food science.

Personally I have benefitted from these books as have my patients. Despite being a marathon runner, for the past 15 years I had a body mass index of 26 and a 36-inch waist (I had a 32-inch waist my first 15 years of adult life, and a 34-inch waist the second 15 years). I enjoyed bread and whole grain cereals. Three months after giving up wheat my waist is 33 inches and I lost 15 pounds with a body mass index of 22. Interestingly, the emerging rosacea on my nose went away. My patients that become wheat free and do not replace wheat with other starches report similar weight loss and health benefits. And, I am now drinking almond milk.

One mistake I now find in this book review is my statement that Perlmutter was wrong to promote saturated fat. I later learned that he was right and I was wrong.

I used my new knowledge of the role of carbohydrates in obesity and the health problems caused by gluten to summarize recent research articles for the publication *Internal Medicine Alert*. Those articles are reprinted here:

The Obesity Epidemic and How We Got It Wrong

Internal Medicine Alert
June 29, 2014;36(12):89-90

Synopsis: There are now 2.1 billion overweight and obese people in the world, up from 857 million people in 1980. The epidemic is global and the U.S. leads the increase among developed countries. This rise coincided with many factors including the development of low fat foods, thinking that saturated fat was the main dietary problem. Recent evidence suggests that the ingestion of high glycemic carbohydrates is the main problem with overweight and obesity and intake of these products increased after the introduction of low fat foods. Grain based starches have among the highest glycemic index even exceeding that of table sugar.

Source: Ng M, Fleming T, Robinson M, et al. Global, regional, and national prevalence of overweight and obesity in children and adults during 1980-2013: A systematic analysis for the Global Burden of Disease Study 2013. The Lancet. 2014; 10.1016/S0140-6736 (14)60460-8. [Epub ahead of print].

The numbers are startling. Worldwide the rates of overweight and obesity have soared in the last 33 years according to the Global Burden of Disease Study 2013, funded by the Bill and Melinda Gates Foundation in cooperation with the World Health Organization. Over half of the obese people live in 10 countries: The USA, China, India, Russia, Brazil, Mexico, Egypt, Germany, Pakistan and Indonesia, showing that obesity is no longer tied to culture or socioeconomic status. There has been a 28% increase overweight and obesity in adults and a 47% increase in children. This robust study looks at both gender and age with respect to rates of overweight and obesity among different countries.

Commentary

Many factors converge to cause overweight and obesity. Most populations have become more sedentary, with increased urbanization. More people eat away from home than previously, especially at "fast food" restaurants. Interestingly, the rise in overweight and obesity starting in the 1980s coincided with the recognition that elevated blood cholesterol is a cardiac risk factor and the development of a low fat food industry.

Thinking that fats, especially saturated fats, are a risk factor for heart disease is logical but is not borne out by the data[1,2]. In his popular book, *Grain Brain*, neurologist and nutritionist David Perlmutter, lays out the benefits of saturated fats, especially on the neurologic system, and describes the dangers of elevated blood sugar coming from ingesting high glycemic carbohydrates[3].

Body fat, especially around the trunk, is associated with hyperlipidemia and the other components of the metabolic syndrome, raising cardiovascular risk. The foods that are most associated with increasing body fat are the high glycemic carbohydrates. Cardiologist William Davis lays out this data well in his popular book, *Wheat Belly*[4].

The glycemic index of foods is a nutritional measure of how much the blood sugar rises in the 90 to 120 minutes after a food is consumed. This measure was developed in a study at the University of Toronto published in 1981[5]. Pure glucose has a glycemic index of 100. Interestingly grain based starches have a higher glycemic index than table sugar[6]. Whole grain bread has a glycemic index of 72, white bread 68, wheat cereal 67 and table sugar 59[4-6].

High glycemic foods trigger rapid insulin release and ultimately the conversion and storage of body fat in persons who are not working or exercising vigorously. High glycemic carbohydrates also drive hunger as rising and falling blood sugars trigger the desire to eat. Replacing fat with carbohydrates, especially grain based foods, has coincided with an increase in calories consumed[7].

Thirty years of discouraging saturated fats and promoting whole grains has been misguided. It is not just about calories in and calories out. The hormonal responses to the calories we eat play a major role in how much we eat and what happens in our body. The problem is excess body fat, especially in the trunk. The nutritional approach to curbing overweight and obesity is to reduce the foods that contribute most to appetite and body fat, and those are the high glycemic carbohydrates, especially grain based foods.

References

1. Chowdhury R, Warnakula S, Kunutsor S, et al. Association of dietary, circulating, and supplement fatty acids with coronary risk; A systemic review. Ann Int Med. 2014;160(6):398-406.
2. Siri-Tarino PW, Sun Q, Hu FB, et al. Meta-analysis of prospective cohort studies evaluating the association of saturated fat with cardiovascular disease. Am J Clin Nutr. 2010;91(3):535-546.
3. Perlmutter D. Grain Brain. New York: Little, Brown and Co. 2013.
4. Davis W. Wheat Belly. New York: Rodale. 2011.
5. Jenkins, DJH, Wolever TM, Taylor RH, et al. Glycemic index of foods: a physiological basis for carbohydrate exchange. Am J Clin Nutr. 1981;34(3):362-366.
6. Juntunen KS, Niskanen LK, Liukkonen KH, et al. Postprandial glucose, insulin and incretin responses to grain products in healthy subjects. Am J Clin Nutr. 2002;75(2):254-262.
7. Jakobsen MU, Dethlefsen C, Joensen AM, at al. Intake of carbohydrates compared with intake of saturated fatty acids and the risk of myocardial infarction: Importance of the glycemic index. Am J Clin Nutr. 2010;91:1764-1768.

Does Gluten Cause Health Problems in Patients Without Celiac Disease?

Internal Medicine Alert
August 29, 2014;36(16):123-124

Synopsis: Gluten is a protein complex that may be inflammatory to humans and is increasingly recognized as a possible cause of numerous health problems such as irritable bowel syndrome, fibromyalgia, skin conditions, allergies, auto-immune arthritis and neurodegenerative conditions.

Source: Volta U, Bardella MT, Calabro A, Troncone R, Corazza GR, et al. An Italian prospective multicenter survey on patients suspected of having non-celiac gluten sensitivity. BMC Med. 2014;12:85.

These Italian investigators enlisted 38 clinical sites (27 adult gastroenterology, 5 internal medicine, 4 pediatrics and 2 allergy) to distribute a questionnaire aimed at identifying patients with health problems possibly associated with non-celiac gluten sensitivity. 486 patients were identified over a one year period, most were female and the mean age was 38 years.

The clinical symptoms associated with gluten were a variety of gastrointestinal complaints: abdominal pain, bloating, diarrhea and/or constipation, nausea, epigastric pain, GERD and aphthous stomatitis. Other complaints included fatigue, fibromyalgia, headache, joint and muscle pain, "foggy mind", dermatitis or skin rash, depression and anxiety. The most frequent diagnoses in these patients were irritable bowel syndrome (47%), food intolerance (35%) and IgE mediated allergy (22%). The time lag between ingestion of gluten and the symptoms varied from a few hours to one day. Diagnostic tests for celiac disease were negative in these patients and those who underwent duodenal biopsy showed normal intestinal mucosa.

The authors conclude that non-celiac gluten sensitivity appears to be associated with a large number of health problems.

Commentary

Non-celiac gluten sensitivity is still medically undefined, but is emerging as a possible probable cause of multiple health problems. Dr. William Davis brought this to light with his 2011 book *Wheat Belly*[1]. Since then there have been multiple reports of remission of conditions with the elimination of gluten, and their relapse when gluten is ingested[2-7]. This area remains very controversial and is criticized by many leading food science centers.

Gluten is not a distinct chemical, but a protein complex consisting of two types of proteins, gliadins and glutenins. Measurement of antibodies to these proteins is used to diagnose celiac disease. Patients with non-gluten sensitivity usually have negative tests for celiac so the diagnosis requires food elimination and clinical judgment. Like other nutritional conditions, using the food, withdrawing it and using it again has diagnostic validity.

William Davis describes in detail how modern wheat is much different than the original wheat used before 1950[1]. Through hybridization, wheat has become much more energy dense with 42 chromosomes compared with the 14 chromosomes of ancient einkorn wheat.

The number of clinical conditions associated with gluten ingestion is staggering. The strongest evidence seems to be with GI distress, skin conditions (my rosacea went away when I stopped gluten and comes back if I ingest it), allergies and fibromyalgia. If these associations are borne out by controlled studies, the burden of disease could be markedly reduced. It is not clear how much of the population is gluten sensitive. The Italian study questionnaire was positive for a small percentage of patients, similar to the prevalence of celiac disease (around 2%). However the real incidence is likely much higher. The association of chronic gluten ingestion and neurodegenerative conditions such as multiple sclerosis, Parkinson's disease and other tremor, and even Alzheimer's disease is alarming[8]. These are described briefly by William Davis[1] and in more detail by neurologist Dr. David Perlmutter in his book, *Grain Brain* [9].

As we learn more about the power of nutrition and the intestinal microbiome, a new area of clinical medicine is opening up. NIH does not have an institute solely devoted to nutritional research, something that nutrition experts regret[10]. I am finding that the longer I am in medicine, the more I follow the words of Hippocrates, "Let food be thy medicine and medicine be thy food".

References

1. Davis W. Wheat Belly. New York: Rodale, 2011.
2. Isasi C, Colmenero I, Casco F, et al. Fibromyalgia and non-celiac gluten sensitivity: a description with

remission of fibromyalgia. Rheumatol Int. 2014;April 12 (Epub ahead of print).

3. Carroccio A, Volta U, Petrolini N, et al. Autoimmune enteropathy and colitis in an adult patient. Dig Dis Sci. 2003;48:1600-1606.
4. Volta U, De Giorgio. New understanding of gluten sensitivity. Nat Rev Gastroenterol Hepatol 2012;9:295-299.
5. Anonymous patient, Rostami K, Hogg-Kollars S, Non-coeliac gluten sensitivity. BMJ 2012;345:e7982.
6. Sapone A, Bai JC, Ciacci C, et al. Spectrum of gluten-related disorders: consensus on new nomenclature and classification. BMC Medicine 2012;10:13.
7. Isasi C, Fernandez-Puga N, Serrano-Vela JI. Fibromyalgia and chronic fatigue syndrome caused by non-celiac gluten sensitivity. Rheumatol Clin. 2014; July 18 (Epub ahead of print).
8. Hadjivassiliou M, Sanders DS, Grunewald RA, et al. Gluten sensitivity; from gut to brain. Lancet. 2010;9:318-330.
9. Perlmutter D, Grain Brain. New York; Little Brown, 2013.
10. Campbell TC, Jacobson H. Whole: Rethinking the Science of Nutrition. Dallas: BenBella, 2013.

My first year on this new nutrition had me about 90% compliant and feeling much healthier. I felt like I had turned back the clock by a decade and my running times demonstrated that. My half marathon times had been over 2 hours from my early 50s to age 63 and now were back under 2 hours. My marathon times have improved by 20 minutes.

I continued to read books on the new nutrition and it was clear I should go 100% into low carbohydrate living and that story is covered next.

PART 3: THE SCIENCE OF LOW CARBOHYDRATE LIVING AND PERFORMANCE

Reading and learning more about healthy nutrition intensified my commitment to a healthy diet of whole foods and being free of grains and low carbohydrate intake daily. They may sound difficult or complicated but it is not. I just follow simple rules of not eating grains, avoiding cow's milk (will still put half and half in coffee), and limiting carbohydrates. The amount of foods available is abundant and no dieting such as calorie counting is involved. By age 65 my waist was back to the 32 inches I enjoyed as a young man in my 20s. That feels great and my running and hiking require much less effort. The next phase of my journey took me deeper into the science.

Jeff Volek is an academic nutrition scientist at The Ohio State University. Has an RD (Registered Dietician) and PhD in nutrition. Stephen Phinney is a physician with a PhD in nutrition and recently retired from the University of California, Davis. Together they have written two recent and very important books, *The Art and Science of Low Carbohydrate Living* (2011) and *The Art and Science of Low*

Carbohydrate Performance (2012). They provide the science behind the work started by Robert Atkins in the 1960s.

The Robert Atkins story is most interesting. It all began with a small study done at the University of Wisconsin and published in the Journal of the American Medical Association (JAMA) in 1963. After reading the two books by Volek and Phinney, I went back and read the 1972 book, *Dr. Atkin's Diet Revolution.* I was amazed by how much of the science of low carbohydrate nutrition was there. Dr. Atkins improved his description of his diet in his 1992 and subsequent editions of *Dr. Atkins New Diet Revolution.*

I wrote an article about the life and courage of Robert Atkins, and could not find a journal willing to publish it. So here it is:

Profile in Courage – Robert Atkins

November, 2014 – Unpublished

That which seems the height of absurdity in one generation often becomes the height of wisdom in another.
John Stuart Mill[1]

Like many physicians educated in the 1970s and for three decades after, I thought Robert Atkins was a kook. As the data accumulated that high cholesterol was a major risk factor for heart disease, and that eating saturated fat most likely contributed to this problem, how dare a physician recommend a diet high in saturated fat and low in the whole grains that provided fiber and other nutrients.

Whatever weight loss that happened on an Atkins diet must be water and temporary, and the diet must be unhealthy.

Recent research is proving Atkins was largely correct. Carbohydrates are the main driver of excess body fat and the changes in the lipids that increase cardiovascular risk[2-7]. Carbohydrates drive hunger by raising insulin levels and causing wide variations in blood sugar. Replacing fat with carbohydrates, especially grain based foods, has coincided with an increase in calories consumed[6].

Eating saturated fat increases satiety and provides sustained energy, increases lean body mass and ultimately results in lower body fat[4,5]. Body fat, especially in the trunk, is the primary lesion of the metabolic syndrome risk factors and is increased through high carbohydrate intake[5,7].

The background of Robert Atkins is both ordinary and impressive. He was born in Columbus, Ohio in 1930 and at the age of 12 the family moved to Dayton. They owned several restaurants. His undergraduate degree was from the University of Michigan. He attended Cornell University Medical College (now Weill Cornell Medical College). After an internship at Strong Hospital in Rochester, NY, he completed his internal medicine residency and fellowship in cardiology at Columbia University. He opened a medical practice in the Upper East Side of Manhattan in 1959[8].

The Atkins diet did not originate with him. In 1963, at age 33, Dr. Atkins was morbidly obese at 224 lbs. and saw a triple chin in the mirror. He read an article in JAMA that advocated a low carbohydrate diet and marked increase in both protein and fat[9]. Atkins found rapid success on this eating plan and began to advocate it for his patients, with equal success. Atkins appeared on The Tonight Show in 1965 and Vogue magazine published his eating plan in 1970 and his diet was originally known as "the Vogue Diet"[8].

Robert Atkins published his groundbreaking book, *Dr. Atkins' Diet Revolution,* in 1972 just as the low fat recommendations were being established and a low fat food industry developed[10]. Ironically, the American Medical Association Council on Nutrition publishing in JAMA condemned the diet that Atkins had developed from a JAMA article 10 years earlier[11]. Americans bought into the low fat food paradigm and Atkins was to be dismissed by the scientific community for decades up to his accidental death from head trauma in 2003.

Thomas Kuhn observed that "normal science" is predicated on the assumption that the scientific community knows what the world is like, and scientists take great pains to defend those assumptions. Scientists tend to ignore research findings that might threaten the existing paradigm and trigger the development of new and competing beliefs. Changing a scientific paradigm only happens through discovery brought on by repeated encounters with anomaly[12]. That is now happening as we shift from low fat to low carbohydrate diet recommendations based on the mounting evidence of the harm of eating a high carbohydrate diet and the benefits of eating more fat than carbohydrate[2-7].

Did Atkins promote the reckless consumption of unhealthy foods? No. I combed his 1972 book for excessive and unhealthy fats. He refers to his diet as steak plus salad plus. While he called for zero carbohydrates, he promoted vegetables and some fruits. What he meant was zero consumption of sugars and refined starches[10]. Ahead of his time, Atkins referred to type 2 diabetes and other hyperglycemia as "carbohydrate intolerance", a term that is being promoted today[5]. In 1972 he described insulin resistance and how high blood sugars result in increased fat deposition[10].

I was in medical school when his first book came out and was taught that the presence of ketones in the blood or urine meant starvation or acidosis. Having ketones in the blood and urine reflects the burning of fat, the best source of sustained energy. Atkins promoted a ketogenic diet to lose weight, something that is being highly recommended by nutrition scientists today, even for high performance athletes[13].

Atkins' 1992 book and two subsequent editions up to 2002 were equally popular and showed his diet was not a fad[14]. The updates here were an embrace of "controlled" carbohydrate eating with more vegetables and some fruits. He advocated the use of the glycemic index of carbohydrates developed at the University of Toronto in 1981[15]. Atkins actively promoted the intake of foods we consider "superfoods" today: spinach, broccoli, kale and berries.

There is room for criticism in the work of Robert Atkins. Despite establishing a multimillion dollar operation, he failed to do research in any meaningful way. He started to promote supplements without an evidence base, and had the conflict of starting his own company that sold nutraceuticals. It became apparent that the later editions of his "Diet Revolution" books were written by a committee with variable quality and making the diet approach more complicated.

These problems and Atkins death in 2003 opened the door for new low carbohydrate diet programs. Another cardiologist, Arthur Agatston, brought forward the widely successful South Beach Diet in 2003[16]. Agatston started work in weight loss in the 1990s and altered the Atkins approach by further differentiating "good carbs" from "bad carbs" based on the glycemic index and "good fats" from "bad fats" based on promoting unsaturated fats over saturated fats. Agatston promoted the South Beach Diet as more "heart healthy" than the Atkins Diet. Today's exoneration of saturated fats calls into question whether the Atkins' Diet was actually less heart healthy than the South Beach Diet.

Currently low carbohydrate diets are gaining wide favor. Another cardiologist, William Davis, has simplified the approach in his book *Wheat Belly* calling for the elimination of all flour based foods, especially wheat that also has the inflammatory protein complex gluten[7]. I lost 20 pounds in 4 months and optimized my weight, body fat, blood sugar and lipids using this simple approach, and it has worked very well with my patients. The current Paleo Diet accomplishes the same goal by eliminating the high glycemic flour based and processed foods[17,18].

Three nutrition scientists, two are physicians at major academic centers, provide a large body of research in favor of the Atkins diet, using of the themes of "the right carbs in the right amounts", "the power of protein", and "meet your new friend: fat"[19]. A recent randomized controlled trial of low carbohydrate versus low fat nutrition expanded the data in favor of low carb by showing that eating more fat and less carbs not only reduces body fat, but also reduces inflammatory markers including small LDL particle size, and increases lean body mass. Eating more carbohydrates and less fat causes the opposite unhealthy effects[2].

Walter Willett of the Harvard School of Public Health has been vocal that fat is not the problem and evidence does not support the recommendation against eating less saturated fat, and that excess carbohydrates are to blame for obesity, diabetes and other metabolic diseases[20,21]. With a similar message, David Perlmutter is lecturing widely after his 2013 book *Grain Brain*[22]. Mark Hyman of The Daniel Plan has been hired by the Cleveland Clinic to lead a Functional Medicine Institute[23,24].

Many nutrition questions remain. What about cancer? If cardiovascular disease is reduced by a low carbohydrate diet, premature death from cancer and other diseases likely affected by nutrition may increase. The generous animal protein advocated by Atkins may still be unhealthy particularly as animals are fed from grain rather than grass. Those advocating a whole food plant based diet have the strongest data to support cancer prevention[25,26]. The power of nutrition is much greater than given credit in medical education and medical research. May the debates begin between the vegan and Paleo diets through further studies.

While Atkins made millions from his books, he was ostracized from his profession. For decades his work came up against the recommendations of scientific authorities, government bodies and organizations such as the American Heart Association (AHA). Now that low carbohydrate eating is rapidly gaining favor, Atkins' name still remains tarnished. It is politically correct to say that you are recommending a "modified" Atkins diet. It is time we gave Robert Atkins the respect he deserves for being a pioneer in combating overweight and obesity.

References

1. Quoted in Stevenson AE. Call to Greatness. Harper, 1954.
2. Bazzano LA, Hu T, Reynolds K, et al. Effects of Low-Carbohydrate and Low-Fat Diets: A Randomized Trial. Ann Intern Med. 2014;161:309-318.
3. Chowdhury R, Warnakula S, Kunutsor S, et al. Association of dietary, circulating, and supplement fatty acids with coronary risk; A systemic review. Ann Int Med. 2014;160(6):398-406.
4. Siri-Tarino PW, Sun Q, Hu FB, et al. Meta-analysis of prospective cohort studies evaluating the association of saturated fat with cardiovascular disease. Am J Clin Nutr. 2010;91(3):535-546.
5. Volek JS, Phinney SD. The Art and Science of Low Carbohydrate Living. Beyond Obesity, LLC. 2011.
6. Jakobsen MU, Dethlefsen C, Joensen AM, at al. Intake of carbohydrates compared with intake of saturated fatty acids and the risk of myocardial infarction: Importance of the glycemic index. Am J Clin Nutr. 2010;91:1764-1768.
7. Davis W. Wheat Belly. Rodale. 2011.
8. Wikipedia, Robert Atkins. Accessed September 30, 2014.
9. Gordon ES, Goldberg M, Chosy GJ. A New Concept in the Treatment of Obesity. JAMA. 1963;186(1):156-166.

10. Atkins RC. Dr. Atkins' Diet Revolution. Bantam Books. 1972.
11. American Medical Association Council on Foods and Nutrition. A Critique of Low-Carbohydrate Ketogenic Weight Reduction Regimens: A Review of Dr. Atkins' Diet Revolution. JAMA. 1973;224:1415-1419.
12. Kuhn TS. The Structure of Scientific Revolutions. University of Chicago Press. 1962.
13. Volek JS, Phinney SD. The Art and Science of Low Carbohydrate Performance. Beyond Obesity, LLC. 2012.
14. Atkins RC. Dr. Atkins' New Diet Revolution. Harper. 1992, 1999, 2002.
15. Jenkins, DJH, Wolever TM, Taylor RH, et al. Glycemic index of foods: a physiological basis for carbohydrate exchange. Am J Clin Nutr. 1981;34(3):362-366.
16. Agatston A. The South Beach Diet. St. Martin's Press. 2003.
17. Voegtlin WL. The Stone Age Diet. Vantage Press, 1975.
18. Cordain L. The Paleo Diet. John Wiley & Sons, 2002, 2011.
19. Westman EC, Phinney SD, Volek JS. The New Atkins for a New You. Touchstone. 2010.
20. Willett WC. Eat, Drink, and Be Healthy: The Harvard Medical School Guide to Healthy Eating. Free Press. Simon & Schuster, 2005.
21. O'Connor A. A Call for a Low-Carb Diet That Embraces Fat. New York Times. September 1, 2014.
22. Perlmutter D. Grain Brain. Little, Brown and Co. 2013.

23. Warren R, Amen D, Hyman M. The Daniel Plan: 40 Days to a Healthier Life. Zondervan, 2013.
24. Townsend A. Cleveland Clinic to open Center for Functional Medicine; Dr. Mark Hyman to be director. Cleveland Plain Dealer. www.cleveland.com/healthfit/index.ssf/2014/09/cleveland_clinic_to_open/cente.html
25. Campbell TC, Jacobson H. Whole: Rethinking the Science of Nutrition. BenBella Books, 2013.
26. Forks Over Knives. Virgil Films Entertainment, 2011. www.youtube.com/user/ForksOverKnives

Wanting to contribute to the literature on low carbohydrate nutrition I reworked the article and the following was published in *The San Diego Physician.*

Overweight and Obesity – It's the Carbohydrates

San Diego Physician
2015;102(4):6-10

The awareness that a low carbohydrate diet rich in protein and saturated fat resulted in a lower body weight has a long history. In 1927 nutritionist Gayelord Hauser came to Hollywood and helped Greta Garbo, Marlene Dietrich and other stars stay lean by avoiding sugars and foods made with flour. Hauser published 19 books between 1930 and 1963 with the most famous being *Look Younger, Live Longer* (1950)[1].

In 1963 the Journal of the American Medical Association (JAMA) published an article from the University of Wisconsin on a novel low carbohydrate diet that achieved rapid weight loss[2]. A young obese Manhattan cardiologist named Robert Atkins read the article and tried the diet. He lost his excess weight rapidly and began using it with patients with great success. Atkins appeared on The Tonight Show in 1965 and Vogue magazine did a story on the diet and it became known as the "Vogue diet" in the 1960s[3]. In 1972 Atkins published his first "Diet Revolution" book and the very low carbohydrate diet rich in fats and protein become known as the Atkins diet[4]. Other popular diets followed calling themselves a "modified Atkins", such as The South Beach Diet in 2003[5].

Meanwhile, in the 1970s mainstream medicine realized that lipids were an important risk factor for cardiovascular disease, the top killer in the industrialized world. By a leap of faith and rational thinking more than good science, the mainstream nutrition and medical community blamed dietary saturated fat for causing high cholesterol and launched new recommended diet programs of less fat and more carbohydrates, especially complex carbohydrates such as "healthy whole grains". Starting in 1980, the overweight and obesity epidemic took off with exponential rises in these conditions over the next three decades.

Recent research is showing that the low carbohydrate diet is largely correct for maintaining a healthy weight[6-10]. Carbohydrates are the main driver of excess body fat by causing fluctuations in blood sugar that increase appetite. Increasing blood sugar causes insulin secretion that drives sugar into cells. What is not burned for energy or stored in the muscles and liver becomes stored fat through lipogenesis. Body fat is hormonally active and causes the four problems of the metabolic syndrome: dyslipidemia, elevated blood sugar, elevated blood pressure and overweight/obesity. There is a genetic contribution to all this but the ill effects of carbohydrate intake beyond our energy needs are universal. Excess sugar converted into fat storage reduces LDL particle size and stimulates inflammatory changes in blood vessels leading to atherosclerosis[6]. Replacing fat with carbohydrates, especially grain based foods, has coincided with an increase in calories consumed[9,10]. Carbohydrates are best obtained from vegetables and whole fruits. Eating more saturated fat and protein reduces hunger and results in fewer calories consumed, the key to the success of low carbohydrate diets.

Two academic nutrition scientists, Jeff Volek, PhD, RD, and Stephen Phinney, MD, PhD, have gathered the science around the low carbohydrate diet in their book for professionals, *The Art and Science of Low Carbohydrate Living*[9]. Their work and others have vindicated the approach taken by Robert Atkins that saturated fat should be a mainstay of a healthy diet. Eating saturated fat from natural sources such as tree nuts, avocados, eggs, meat and fish reduces hunger and overall calorie intake resulting lower body fat.

Volek and Phinney have also triggered a trend among high performance endurance athletes to move away from carbohydrate loading and sweetened energy drinks. They show that a ketogenic diet of steady fat burning will improve performance over burning a temporary supply of carbohydrates[11]. Humans are not like hybrid cars readily able to convert from one energy source to another, in our case from carbohydrate to fat burning. If athletes depend on carbs for energy, there is a drop in energy and muscle cramps when they run out. No more pasta before events, eat the steak! Drink water rather than sweet energy drinks and gels and get necessary salt, fat and protein during long events such as a marathons and ultramarathons, triathlons, bicycle races and hiking.

Men's professional tennis is a grueling sport especially in major events that can go to 5 sets and over 4 hours. Of the leading male tennis professionals, Novak Djokovic follows a very low carbohydrate diet and relies on fat burning during performances[12]. Interestingly in the 2015 Australian Open, the semi-final had Djokovic facing defending champion Stan Wawrinka in a match that went 5 sets. The score in the final set was Djokovic 6-0. In the final Djokovic faced Brad Murray in a 4 set match. The score in the final set was Djokovic 6-0. What role did diet play in this success with endurance?

My story is revealing. I started running marathons at age 29 and was lean and fit with a 32-inch waist. I stopped running long distances after a few years and as someone who loved breads and muffins, my waist increased to 36 inches and my weight went to 192 from about 160. At age 46 my total cholesterol was 211 and my HDL cholesterol was only 37. I returned to running marathons and was able to get my weight down to 180 with a total cholesterol of 175 and an HDL of 52. I was happy but my waist was still 36. At age 62 I read *Wheat Belly* by Dr. William Davis and gave up the grains. In four months my weight was 160, my waist 32 and my total cholesterol was 152 with an HDL of 69. I am running marathons and half marathons faster than any time in 10 years. Best yet I feel much younger and have very little of the old appetite and stay awake and alert in the afternoon and even during an evening symphony.

The dominant cause and solution to the overweight and obesity epidemic remains hidden in plain sight – it's the carbohydrates. The food industry flourishes on selling foods made with flour and sugar. These food commodities are the easiest to package and store, and hence result in greater profits. The food industry also funds major health organizations, nutritional research institutes and federal agencies that provide dietary recommendations, resulting in much inertia to change[13,14].

Countering the status quo of boxes of high carbohydrate foods lining our supermarket aisles is a growing worldwide realization that eating the food that nature has provided for millions of years is better for us than the more recent breads and processed foods. The Paleo Diet was introduced in 1975 and is becoming a new fashion whether people understand the nutrition behind it or not[15,16]. French physician Pierre Dukan has been promoting a low carbohydrate diet for over 30 years and the Dukan Diet is increasingly popular in Great Britain and France[17].

Walter Willett of the Harvard School of Public Health has been vocal that fat is not the problem and evidence does not support the recommendation against eating less saturated fat, and that excess carbohydrates are to blame for obesity, diabetes and other metabolic diseases[20,21]. A growing number of physician innovators that are using the evidence about carbohydrates to educate the public, include William Davis[12,18], David Perlmutter[19] and Mark Hyman, nutrition advisor to Bill Clinton and recently hired by the Cleveland Clinic to lead a new Functional Medicine Institute[20].

Paradigm changes in science and medicine happen slowly. Thomas Kuhn observed that "normal science" is predicated on the assumption that the scientific community knows what the world is like, and scientists take great pains to defend those assumptions. Scientists tend to ignore research findings that might threaten the existing paradigm and trigger the development of new and competing beliefs. Changing a scientific paradigm only happens through discovery brought on by repeated encounters with anomaly[21]. The paradigm around what is a healthy diet is changing from low fat to a low carbohydrate diet rich in natural fats and proteins.

References

1. Gayelord Hauser. Widipedia.org. Accessed February 5, 2015.
2. Gordon ES, Goldberg M, Chosy GJ. A New Concept in the Treatment of Obesity. JAMA. 1963;186(1):156-166.
3. Wikipedia, Robert Atkins. Accessed February 5, 2015.
4. Atkins RC. Dr. Atkins' Diet Revolution. Bantam Books. 1972.
5. Agatston A. The South Beach Diet. St. Martin's Press. 2003.
6. Bazzano LA, Hu T, Reynolds K, et al. Effects of Low-Carbohydrate and Low-Fat Diets: A Randomized Trial. Ann Intern Med. 2014;161:309-318.
7. Chowdhury R, Warnakula S, Kunutsor S, et al. Association of dietary, circulating, and supplement fatty acids with coronary risk; A systemic review. Ann Int Med. 2014;160(6):398-406.

8. Siri-Tarino PW, Sun Q, Hu FB, et al. Meta-analysis of prospective cohort studies evaluating the association of saturated fat with cardiovascular disease. Am J Clin Nutr. 2010;91(3):535-546.
9. Volek JS, Phinney SD. The Art and Science of Low Carbohydrate Living. Beyond Obesity, LLC. 2011.
10. Jakobsen MU, Dethlefsen C, Joensen AM, at al. Intake of carbohydrates compared with intake of saturated fatty acids and the risk of myocardial infarction: Importance of the glycemic index. Am J Clin Nutr. 2010;91:1764-1768.
11. Volek JS, Phinney SD. The Art and Science of Low Carbohydrate Performance. Beyond Obesity, LLC. 2012.
12. Davis W. Wheat Belly. Rodale. 2011.
13. Campbell TC, Jacobson H. Whole: Rethinking the Science of Nutrition. BenBella Books, 2013.
14. Minger D. Death By Food Pyramid. Primal Blueprint Publishing, 2013.
15. Voegtlin WL. The Stone Age Diet. Vantage Press, 1975.
16. Cordain L. The Paleo Diet. John Wiley & Sons, 2002, 2011.
17. Dukan Diet. Wikipedia.org, Accessed February 18, 2015.
18. Davis W. Wheat Belly Total Health, Rodale, 2014.
19. Perlmutter D. Grain Brain. Little, Brown and Co. 2013.
20. Townsend A. Cleveland Clinic to open Center for Functional Medicine; Dr. Mark Hyman to be director. Cleveland Plain Dealer. www.cleveland.com/healthfit/index.ssf/2014/09/cleveland_clinic_to_open/cente.html

21. Kuhn TS. The Structure of Scientific Revolutions. University of Chicago Press. 1962.

Low carbohydrate nutrition and athletic performance is a revolutionary development and demonstrates that carbohydrate loading and carbohydrate energy drinks and gels are a mistake for athletes needing to perform for hours. As Volek and Phinney describe, with the data to support it, we can only store limited carbohydrate energy. On the other hand, even with a very low body fat, we store much more fat energy, a difference of 2000 calories of carbohydrate energy compared with 80,000 calories of fat energy. If we load up with carbohydrates, we will preferentially burn that until it is depleted. We are not as efficient as hybrid cars able to readily switch from one energy source to another. When we deplete our carbohydrates we get muscle cramps and feel dizzy.

If we follow a low carbohydrate diet, such as not more than 50 grams of carbohydrate daily from natural foods, we become a fat burner. This transition in our body takes a few months to develop. Once it happens, we can perform for many hours with a stable blood sugar and no drop in energy. We become ketogenic (ketones are the breakdown products of fat) using our tremendous stores of fat energy as our fuel from the beginning.

The top in the world tennis player, Novak Djokovic, credits a low carbohydrate diet for his success. If you look at his scores in winning long matches, he usually wins the final set handily. He is still full of energy while his opponents become carbohydrate depleted and exhausted. As I write this, the U.S. Open tennis tournament is underway and despite fine weather, large numbers of players are cramping up and withdrawing from their matches. The high carbohydrate snacks cannot keep them going.

I experienced this effect in my marathon running, and follow a low carbohydrate diet. With no carbohydrate loading and avoiding carbs at the rest stops, instead having some fat and protein such as from dark chocolate and nuts, and drinking only water, I just keep going. I am now able to sprint over the finish line with better times.

The science behind low carbohydrate nutrition has a long history but remains hidden in plain sight. It is a revolution for nutrition science and a paradigm change for how most Americans eat. As Thomas Kuhn describes in his classic 1962 book, *The Structure of Scientific Revolutions,* paradigms only change after many exposures to new findings. Scientists tend to ignore information that does not fit their paradigm until they can no longer ignore the new knowledge. Also with nutrition, there are powerful forces against changing away from carbohydrates. Grains are the most profitable food commodity and billions of dollars are at stake.

The complexities of the economics and politics of the food industry are well described by Colin Campbell in his book, *Whole: Rethinking the Science of Nutrition* (2013) and by Denise Minger in *Death by Food Pyramid* (2014).

As I became fully devoted to low carbohydrate eating, I enjoy the health benefits of a constant clear headedness. I also believe that I have reduced my risks of the chronic diseases that plague us as we age, hopefully avoiding the

Parkinson's disease of my father. My knowledge journey was far from over as I describe in the final part of this book.

JOSEPH E. SCHERGER, MD, MPH

PART 4: TOTAL HEALTH IN BODY AND MIND

"No disease that can be treated by diet should be treated with any other means".
Maimonides

I started this journey to low carbohydrate nutrition two years before this writing by reading William Davis, a cardiologist who reversed his type 2 diabetes and excess body fat by giving up all wheat products, as David Perlmutter, the neurologist described earlier. After these two physicians published their original works, they went on social media and learned from the wisdom of the crowds of people who embrace this nutrition revolution. They also became leaders in a new medical field called functional medicine. Functional medicine seeks to find the root causes of disease and repair that rather than simply treat disease with drugs and procedures.

The excess carbohydrates causing overweight and obesity is straightforward. Carbohydrates create an unstable blood sugar and we become hungry when our blood sugar is falling. The high carbohydrate American diet results in our eating about 30% more calories that we would if we consumed more fats from natural sources (William Davis, *Wheat Belly*).

The impact of the inflammatory proteins of grains on our health is much more complex. This is explored in the second book by William Davis, *Wheat Belly Total Health* (2014). Prolamin proteins such as the gluten complex cause a leaky gut phenomenon where proteins from the intestine never meant for our bloodstream get in and cause an inflammatory immune reaction. In some people with repeated exposure to these proteins an auto-immune condition develops with our own antibodies attacking different organs of our body. The entire range of auto-immune diseases, hypothyroidism, rheumatoid and other inflammatory arthritis conditions, skin diseases such as acne, rosacea and psoriasis, neurological diseases such as multiple sclerosis, may be caused by our nutrition. Most of these diseases are unique to humans and are not found in the animal kingdom eating food from natural sources. The burden of diseases that appear to be caused by this malnutrition is staggering.

David Perlmutter in his second book, *Brain Maker* (2015) brings the early knowledge of the intestinal microbiome into the picture. We have about 100 trillion bacteria in and on our body, 10 times the number of cells, and most of these bacteria are in our gut. They determine our health in ways previously unimagined. These bacteria are completely determined by what we eat, and they change accordingly. A healthy whole food diet results in a healthy microbiome and unhealthy eating, especially inflammatory proteins, causes an unhealthy microbiome and the gut phenomenon described above. Our intestinal bacteria have a direct connection to the health of our brains and an unhealthy microbiome through malnutrition may be the underlying cause of neurodegeneration culminating in Alzheimer's dementia.

I have written book reviews of both of these works published in *Family Medicine* and presented here:

Wheat Belly Total Health

Family Medicine
Accepted, publication pending

William Davis, MD
New York: Rodale, 2014

In his 2011 book, *Wheat Belly,* William Davis presented a new perspective on low carbohydrate nutrition[1]. He argued that the high glycemic index and high glycemic load of grains, especially wheat, were primary drivers of overweight, obesity and type 2 diabetes. The so called "healthy whole wheat" increased hunger though elevated blood sugars and the pouring out of insulin causing people to eat about 30% more calories. In addition, he argued that the inflammatory protein complex gluten in wheat, barley and rye is associated with a large burden of disease in multiple organ systems.

William Davis is a cardiologist practicing near Milwaukee. As he describes in his follow-up book, *Wheat Belly Total Health*, he was obese, had type 2 diabetes and dyslipidemia with an HDL cholesterol of 27. All of this reversed when he gave up eating grains.

After *Wheat Belly,* Davis used social media to create a dialogue on his website, wheatbellyblog.com and on Facebook. He became further educated by the "wisdom of the crowd" and *Wheat Belly Total Health* is the result. It is much denser delving into the principles and practice of functional medicine and their approach to nutrition[2]. All grains become the target and Davis argues that non-gluten seeds of grasses such as oats, corn and rice are as inflammatory to the human body as gluten.

Wheat Belly Total Health is divided into three parts: No grain is a good grain, living grainlessly, and be a grainless overachiever. The clear organization stops there as the text becomes scattered. Problems with the GI tract, nervous system and thyroid are presented multiple times with varying degrees of detail. While *Wheat Belly Total Health* has more nutritional depth than *Wheat Belly,* its lack of coherency makes it a more frustrating read, especially for patients lacking a background in nutrition and inflammatory health problems.

Low carbohydrate and anti-inflammatory nutrition are trends that have mounting scientific evidence, and should be part of the teaching of medical students, residents and physicians in practice. There is now well documented high quality evidence that a low carbohydrate diet is superior to the low fat diet the American Heart Association has recommended for decades[3]. Evidence for the inflammatory effects of gluten in non-celiac patients has accumulated in observational studies from around the world[4,5].

Like other popular books promoting a certain nutrition, Davis exaggerates the evidence. From the beginning of the book, he boasts from a one-sided perspective. There is no expression of humility and little expression of a need for more evidence. Evidence of benefit from grain based fiber is dismissed outright. Despite these limitations the book is important and worth recommending to learners and patients. I recommend reading *Wheat Belly* first as an introduction and then *Wheat Belly Total Health* for a deeper dive into grain free nutrition.

The most valuable parts of *Wheat Belly Total Health* are the explanations of why some people do not lose weight with the elimination of grains. There is a good explanation of thyroid function, especially the conversion of the storage hormone T4 into the active hormone T3 that may be blocked by chronic ingestion of grains. I am now ordering more Free T3 tests with TSH in overweight and obese patients. When the Free T3 is low, an addition of T3 in the treatment may result in rapid weight loss. Deficiencies of iodine and vitamin D are also discussed in detail.

There is a large inconvenient truth emerging in the nutrition science that food many Americans enjoy, bread, cookies, cakes, bagels, and tortillas, are unhealthy. Grains have been hybridized to become much more energy dense than the original forms found in nature. The high glycemic consequences are seen in an overweight and obese society. Coupled with the burden of disease postulated from inflammatory foods, there is much to be said for going grain free. William Davis, along with neurologist David Perlmutter[6,7] and family physician Mark Hyman[8], are committed physician authors grounded in functional medicine and well worth making part of the educational dialogue of nutrition science.

References

1. Davis W. *Wheat Belly*. New York:Rodale, 2011.
2. Institute for Functional Medicine. www.functionalmedicine.org

3. Bazzano LA, Hu T, Reynolds K, et al. Effects of Low-Carbohydrate and Low-Fat Diets: A Randomized Trial. Ann Intern Med. 2014;161:309-318.
4. Hadjivassiliou M, Sanders DS, Grunewald RA, et al. Gluten sensitivity; from gut to brain. Lancet. 2010;9:318-330.
5. Volta U, Bardella MT, Calabro A, Troncone R, Corazza GR, et al. An Italian prospective multicenter survey on patients suspected of having non-celiac gluten sensitivity. BMC Med. 2014;12:85.
6. Perlmutter D. Grain Brain. New York: Little, Brown & Co., 2013.
7. Perlmutter D, Loberg K. Brain Maker. New York: Little, Brown & Co. 2015.
8. Hyman M. The Blood Sugar Solution 10 Day Detox Diet. New York: Little, Brown & Co. 2014.

Brain Maker

Family Medicine
Accepted, publication pending

David Perlmutter, MD with Kristin Loberg
New York: Little, Brown and Co. 2015

You are what you feed your gut microbiome. That is the central message of David Perlmutter's second book on nutrition and the health of the brain. In his first book *Grain Brain* (Little, Brown and Co. 2013), Perlmutter discussed how elevated blood sugar from grains and sweets combined with the inflammatory proteins of grains to cause much of the neurodegenerative conditions afflicting humans including Alzheimer's Disease. In *Brain Maker* Perlmutter brings forth the emerging science on the gut microbiome and how it affects the brain and our overall health.

This is an important book that describes scientifically, with some hyperbole, a new frontier in medicine. The NIH started the Human Microbiome Project in 2008 and what is coming out of this is a whole new organ system affecting human health[1]. While the 100 trillion organisms are segregated in the gut, orifices and the skin, they chemically interact throughout the body. The gut microbiome develops after birth and is completely dependent on what we eat.

Brain Maker is divided into three parts. Part 1 describes the gut microbiome and its impact on health and disease. Whether we are born sterile is not completely known, there may be *in utero* microbiome development, but for the most part our gut microbiome is initiated at birth through the vaginal birth canal. Perlmutter describes the risks involved with Cesarean birth and describes how gauze with vaginal fluids may be applied to a baby's mouth. Breastfeeding is ideal for getting the gut microbiome off to a healthy start.

Part 2 describes what goes wrong. Gluten and fructose, abundant in our common foods, lead to inflammation in the body by negatively impacting the gut microbiome. The proteins of grains, specifically the gluten protein complex, and high fructose corn syrup in sweets, combine to cause inflammatory reactions starting in the gut. The biology of "leaky gut" is described in common language for a public audience but also with solid scientific detail. The leakage of inflammatory proteins from the gut into the bloodstream and their effect on mitochondria set the stage for auto-immune disease.

The information that our gut microbiome affects our mood and may contribute to anxiety and depression is becoming well known[2]. Perlmutter goes much further and makes an impressive case that an unhealthy gut microbiome is the likely cause of Autism Spectrum Disorders. Case reports are included about the reversal of symptoms in Autism and Tourette syndrome that may be accomplished through probiotic enemas and fecal transplantation.

In Part 3 Perlmutter gives his recommendations for developing and maintaining a healthy gut microbiome. He emphasizes fermented foods such as yogurt, kefir and pickled foods as the stars of a good diet. He emphasizes a low carbohydrate, high-quality fat diet and lists the "brain maker foods". He recommends some supplements including probiotics, especially when taking an antibiotic, and DHA, turmeric, coconut oil, alpha-lipoic acid, and vitamin D. Overall Perlmutter does not push supplements as much as he did in *Grain Brain.*

Many people reading this book will feel that Perlmutter goes way too far in his statements and recommendations, and they may be right, but there is new knowledge and therapeutic breakthroughs that will further develop in this new area of science and medicine.

In summary, *Brain Maker* is worth reading and recommending to learners and patients, with some caveats. Perlmutter is daring and the full truth about what he presents will take time but the reader will be impressed with the overall message. I tell patients to focus on Part 3 of the book and bring me their questions. The emergence of knowledge about our gut microbiome makes what we eat even more important to our health. The old expression "you are what you eat" is being modified to include an important intermediary, the gut microbiome.

References

1. NIH Human Microbiome Project. http://hmpdacc.org/
2. Smith PA. Can the Bacteria in Your Gut Explain Your Mood? New York Times, June 23, 2015.

I explored the connection between the gut microbiome and the brain further with this article in *Internal Medicine Alert*:

You Are What You Feed Your Gut Microbiome

Internal Medicine Alert
August 29, 2015;37(16):121-122

Synopsis: The human gut microbiome regulates intestinal function and health. There is mounting evidence that the gut microbiome influences the immune system and the central and peripheral nervous systems. This article reviews the bidirectional relationship between the gut microbiome and brain disorders.

Source: Petra AI, Panagiotidou S, Hatziagelaki E, et al. Gut-Microbiota-Brain Axis and its Effect on

Neuropsychiatric Disorders With Suspected Immune Dysfunction. Clin Ther. 2015;37:984-995.

These authors reviewed articles on Medline starting in 1980 for a wide range of neurologic disorders and two systems, the gut-microbiota-brain axis and the hypothalamic-pituitary-adrenal axis. Bidirectional influences exist between the brain and the gut flora that are associated with mood disorders, autism-spectrum disorders, attention-deficit hypersensitivity disorder, multiple sclerosis and obesity. This article joins a growing list of other studies illuminating these relationships[1-4].

Bacterial dysbiosis, small intestinal bacterial overgrowth, and increased intestinal permeability may produce numerous immunologic effects including central nervous system inflammation. Our mood is affected by these changes. Bacterial proteins cross-react with human antigens to stimulate dysfunctional responses of the immune system that may lead to neurodegenerative disorders.

Communication between the gut and the brain goes both ways. Antibiotics, environmental and infectious agents, intestinal neurotransmitters, sensory vagal fibers, cytokines and essential metabolites all convey information to the central nervous system (CNS) about the intestinal state. The hypothalamic-pituitary-adrenal axis are the CNS regulatory areas of satiety, and neuropeptides released from sensory nerve fibers affect the gut microbiota composition directly or through nutrient availability. Such interactions appear to influence the pathogenesis of a number of nervous system disorders, from mood to auto-immune neurodegenerative conditions to obesity.

Commentary

"You are what you eat" is an age old expression highlighting that we are organisms that depend on food for growth and survival. The title even became a popular diet and TV program in the United Kingdom from 2004-2007. With the emphasis in modern medicine on pharmacologic therapies and procedures, the vital importance of nutrition has been downplayed in human health and disease. Many people eat whatever they want and health care does little to intervene. We continue to have debates on what constitutes a healthy diet.

The recent appreciation of the gut microbiome, the 100 trillion organisms that resides within us, has added a new dimension to this expression. These gut bacteria together weigh about 10 pounds and would occupy a half gallon container. They are a new vital organ to the human species. They completely depend on us for sustenance.

The gut microbiome is an important intermediary between what we eat and our health. The gut bacteria get first crack at what we eat and play a vital role in what gets into our bodies and what happens to these nutrients. A healthy gut microbiome is critical for good health and an unhealthy gut microbiome assures that we will not be well.

The science around the gut microbiome is in its infancy. The Human Microbiome Project at the NIH was established in 2008[5]. The emerging knowledge from this "new organ" is a paradigm shift for medicine. Hopefully it will usher in renewed interest in human nutrition and its impact on our health.

References

1. Galland L. The gut microbiome and the brain. J Med Food. 2014;17:1261-1272.
2. O'Mahony SM, Clarke G, Borre YE, Dinan TG, Cryan JF. Serotonin, tryptophan metabolism and the brain-gut-microbiome axis. Behavioral Brain Research. 2015;277:32-48.
3. Perlmutter D. Brain Maker. New York: Little, Brown and Co. 2015.
4. Mayer EA, Tillisch K, Gupta A. Gut/brain axis and the microbiota. J. Clin Invest. 2015;125:926-938.
5. NIH Human Microbiome Project. http://hmpdacc.org/

Using the knowledge I gained from William Davis and David Perlmutter I realize that we have the opportunity to eliminate many human diseases. This article focuses on diabetes:

Eliminating Diabetes – Diseases of Malnutrition

Desert Health
October, 2015

Diabetes mellitus is a group of diseases that have in common an elevated blood sugar. They are disorders of carbohydrate metabolism. Emerging scientific evidence points to malnutrition, not the starvation type, but rather eating the wrong foods, as the dominant cause of diabetes.

There is a genetic component to developing diabetes, but this is small in comparison to the impact of nutrition. The frequency of diabetes has increased exponentially since 1980 along with the increase in overweight and obesity due to what we eat.

This article describes the impact of what we eat on the development of both type 1 and type 2 diabetes. Diabetes that develops during pregnancy, gestational diabetes, will be lumped with type 2 diabetes because they have essentially the same mechanisms that result in high blood sugar. The information in this article draws mainly from the work of two physicians, William Davis (*Wheat Belly* and *Wheat Belly Total Health*) and David Perlmutter (*Grain Brain* and *Brain Maker*).

As a group, the diseases of diabetes have a tremendous impact on the health of Americans causing heart disease, stroke, organ failure, blindness, neuropathy, dementia and premature death. Collectively we spend more money treating diabetes than any other group of diseases including cancer and heart disease. Eliminating diabetes, or making it very rare, would be an enormous benefit to our collective health. This may seem far-fetched but eliminating diabetes is easily within our reach. All we need to do is to eat the right foods.

Inside the body, the mechanisms of diabetes are highly complex. Drugs used to treat diabetes attempt to manipulate these mechanisms. However, the triggers of diabetes are not complex. Unfortunately, they remain largely hidden in plain sight.

Inflammatory proteins – Auto-immunity – Type 1 Diabetes

Type 1 diabetes is one of many auto-immune diseases that rob us of our health. In the case of type 1 diabetes, we form antibodies that attack and destroy the cells in the pancreas that make insulin. Without insulin we cannot metabolize sugar and we die. All type 1 diabetics must take insulin to live. The complications of type 1 diabetes even treated with insulin include reduced circulation to many parts of the body, blindness, kidney failure, neuropathy and heart disease. Without optimal treatment, people with type 1 diabetes die prematurely.

What causes us to form these auto-antibodies that destroy our own tissues? For years this was thought to be due to viruses that reprogram our DNA. We now know that "leaky gut" from food substances, mainly proteins, get into blood stream and are considered foreign by our immune system. We form antibodies against these proteins, a type of inflammatory reaction, that also attack and destroy our tissues, in this case the insulin-making cells of our pancreas.

Where do these inflammatory proteins come from? Mainly from eating grains such as wheat and other foods made with flour. Grains such wheat and oats contain prolamin proteins, such as the gluten protein complex, that are inflammatory to the human body and increase intestinal permeability or "leaky gut". It appears to be that the entire spectrum of auto-immune disease, hypothyroidism, rheumatoid arthritis and other inflammatory arthritis, multiple sclerosis and other neurodegenerative diseases, and many allergies are the result of eating inflammatory proteins. These diseases are for the most part unique to humans and are not seen in the animal kingdom.

Excess carbohydrates – Increased body fat – Type 2 and Gestational Diabetes

Body fat is much more than the storage of energy. Fat is hormonally active in the body and causes inflammation and changes in carbohydrate metabolism. While genetics play a role in susceptibility, there is a level of body fat that would result in almost everyone developing type 2 diabetes.

What causes increased body fat? We now understand it is not from the fatty foods we eat. In general fats satisfy us and reduce hunger. Increased body fat comes mainly from eating carbohydrates -- grains, sweets and alcohol that drive up hunger and cause us to eat more. Carbohydrates and fat are energy foods and the body will try to use the carbohydrates first. All the excess carbohydrates we consume that are not used for energy are stored as body fat through a mechanism called lipogenesis.

Carbohydrates are sugars and starches and come mainly from grains and sweets. Starches such as grains are simply chains of sugar. The amount of sugar in a carbohydrate food is called the glycemic load. It turns out the grains such as the wheat in bread, muffins, cookies, cakes and pizza crust have the highest glycemic load along with sweets such as ice cream.

During pregnancy women eat much more and if excess carbohydrates are consumed, gestational diabetes is often the result, putting the baby and the mother at risk.

You are what you eat

This old phrase has new meanings now that the gut microbiome, the 100 trillion organisms in our intestines that determine much of our health, is being understood. Eating the whole foods of nature -- nuts, vegetables, fruit, seeds, healthy fish and meat, results in a healthy gut flora and healthy intestines. Diabetes would be very rare if this is all we ate. Inflammatory proteins and excess sugars result in an unhealthy gut flora, leaky gut, inflammation and a staggering burden of disease, including the diseases of diabetes. Stop this malnutrition and we can stop diabetes.

My journey into healthy nutrition and greater wellness is far from over. Life is a journey and I plan to stay active and contribute to the knowledge of wellness as long as I can, which hopefully will be a long time. We have just begun to understand the real impact nutrition has on our health.

EPILOGUE

There are many inconvenient truths facing the human race today. Al Gore gave us greater awareness of the impact of climate change, accelerated by our lack of caring for our planet. Many of our societies have fallen victim to entropy, greater disorganization and violence. The inconvenient truth in nutrition is that we have created a remarkably unhealthy diet. What we thought was healthy for decades turns out to be wrong.

The anthropologist and physiologist (just to name two of his expertise) Jared Diamond declared in 1999 in Discover magazine that becoming farmers was the worst mistake in the history of the human race. Evidence shows that we were much healthier as hunter/gatherers with greater height, stronger bones, and better teeth just to mention a few findings. This truth is the basis for the Paleolitihic Diet (Paleo for short) originally described by gastroenterologist Walter Voegtlin in the 1970s. Loren Cordain made the diet popular in is 2002 book, *The Paleo Diet*.

So far food science at major American universities, heavily funded by the food industry, may have caused us more harm than good. We have genetically modified many foods without regard for the impact on our complex physiology, including the gut microbiome. William Davis goes into detail about modern 42 chromosome wheat engineered by hybridization at the University of Minnesota by Norman Borlag who died a great hero. We are paying the price of the unintended consequences of this wheat compared with the 14 chromosome natural wheat that we probably shouldn't be eating anyway. Food science must become much more sophisticated as it attempts to genetically modify the foods of nature. We do that at our potential benefit and peril.

I continue to speak and write on nutrition and a healthy lifestyle. Amazingly in my 60s my medical practice changed more than any time previous. I plan to stay lean and fit and hope to inspire my patients and readers of this book to do also. We have so much more to learn and have within our power to develop the healthiest humans ever in our 5 million year history.

APPENDICES

Appendix I

Suggested Daily Meal Plan

Healthy nutrition does not require counting calories, even if you want to lose weight. By eating a diet high in fat and protein from healthy sources, the appetite is greatly reduced resulting in eating fewer calories naturally. Limited carbohydrates, and eating only those in natural foods, does not result in the unstable blood sugar common among those eating grains, sweets and drinking excessive alcohol. Here is a typical daily meal plan I follow:

Breakfast

My bowl no longer contains cereal, rather:

1. A handful of tree nuts (almonds, walnuts, pecans, cashew nuts or Brazil nuts) Mix and match as you like for variety.

2. A layer of berries, usually fresh blueberries but sometimes strawberries, raspberries or blackberries, or as back-up dried cranberries. About ¼ cup.
3. Four heaping tablespoons of plain yogurt with live cultures, preferably goat milk or coconut milk. Will settle for cow's milk if that is all that is available. Alternative or in addition some Kefir, another fermented food.
4. A layer of ground flaxseed, chia seeds or hemp seeds.
5. Unsweetened almond milk or coconut milk for added moisture. Will use whole cow's milk if that is all that is available.

Two eggs, hard boiled or fried in olive oil or butter.

After these high protein foods, I may have a banana and/or an orange. The sugar in these fruits is absorbed more slowly after eating protein.

Water, coffee, or tea are the best beverages during the day.

This hearty breakfast will nourish me even with hard work for 5-6 hours.

Lunch

A salad, preferably a spinach salad with other vegetables (especially avocado and tomatoes), nuts, berries and a protein such as shrimp, salmon or chicken breast. No croutons!

Water, coffee or tea.

Dinner

An entrée source of protein such as wild salmon, scallops or other fish. If meat, eat a modest portion of grass fed beef such as a petit filet, lamb, pork, chicken or turkey. I eat fish two times to one over meat.

Healthy vegetables such as garlic spinach, asparagus, broccoli, squash or yams, carrots, and tomatoes. Sometimes natural whole or Rosemary potatoes. Sometimes my dinner is vegetarian with eggplant or tofu as the high protein entrée.

Water and one glass of red wine (other alcohol may be used but avoid the grains such as wheat in beer). An ultra-light beer is acceptable, as is white wine.

A modest amount of dark chocolate may be taken for dessert with the glass of wine. Look for at least 70% cocoa.

This meal plan does not require any snacking, and snacking is to be avoided. If an afternoon snack is desired, I recommend an apple.

Appendix II

Recommended Reading

William Davis, *Wheat Belly* (2011) and *Wheat Belly Total Health* (2014). Both by Rodale.

Dr. Davis is a cardiologist who got me started after I read *Wheat Belly* in 2013 and became free of grains. His books are well referenced and he is the champion of a grain free lifestyle. Dr. Davis reversed his own type 2 diabetes and developed extraordinarily healthy lipids from following this approach to eating. He is a modern day Robert Atkins, another cardiologist who healed himself before healing others.

David Perlmutter, *Grain Brain* (2013) and *Brain Maker* (2015). Both by Little, Brown & Co.

Dr. Perlmutter is a neurologist with an advanced degree in nutrition. *Grain Brain* built off of William Davis *Wheat Belly* and emphasized how high blood sugar and the inflammatory effects of grains cause a host of neurodegenerative diseases including Alzheimer's disease. *Brain Maker* is a breakthrough book bringing the emerging science about the crucial role of the gut microbiome in health and disease, a new "organ" that totally depends on what we eat. An unhealthy gut microbiome, induced by grains, causes leaky gut and most auto-immune diseases and neurodegeneration.

Daniel Lieberman, *The Story of the Human Body: Evolution, Health and Disease* (2013). Vintage Books.

This Harvard evolutionary biologist is a genius and knows more about health, nutrition and disease than the vast majority of physicians. He describes in detail how the nutrition of our Paleolithic ancestors was much healthier than our processed foods today.

Jeff Volek & Stephen Phinney. *The Art and Science of Low Carbohydrate Living* (2011) and *The Art and Science of Low Carbohydrate Performance* (2012). Both by Beyond Obesity, LLC.

Jeff Volek, RD, PhD is an academic nutritionist at The Ohio State University and Stephen Phinney, MD, PhD recently retired from the food science department at the University of California, Davis. They provide the hard science behind the benefits of low carbohydrate nutrition. In their book on performance, they describe how great endurance athletes such as the tennis player, Novak Djokovic excel without eating carbohydrates except for in whole foods. Being a steady fat burner during long athletic events results in a steady blood sugar and steady performance compared with athletes that get tired, dizzy or cramp when they bottom out their limited supply of carbohydrates.

T. Colin Campbell & Howard Jacobson. *Whole: Rethinking the Science of Nutrition* (2013). BenBella Books.

Colin Campbell is a distinguished nutrition scientist at Cornell (now emeritus). His research focused on nutrition and cancer and he conducted the largest epidemiologic research in the world showing that cancer and animal protein are strongly associated. He is a champion of a whole food plant based diet (being vegan). He first published *The China Study* in 2006 and *Whole* summarizes those findings and provides a critique of how most nutrition science falls short in providing the information we need due to attempting to study single nutrients rather than whole foods. He also describes how the food industry in America is suppressing vital information about healthy and unhealthy foods.

Rick Warren, Daniel Amen & Mark Hyman. *The Daniel Plan: 40 Days to a Healthier Life* (2013). Zondervan.

Rick Warren was an overweight pastor in Orange County, CA and decided he had better lose weight and become healthy. Rather than do that by himself he challenged his congregation to join him. He enlisted the help of two physicians, Daniel Amen, a psychiatrist who has shown through imaging studies that the higher the blood sugar the more rapid the brain atrophy, and Mark Hyman, a family physician who advised Bill Clinton on becoming healthier by giving up grains and processed food. This book covers how in 40 days the congregation lost over a hundred thousand pounds. Rick Warren provides spiritual advice while the doctors advise on healthy nutrition.

Denise Minger. *Death by Food Pyramid: How Shoddy Science, Sketchy Politics and Shady Special Interests Have Ruined Our Health... and How to Reclaim It.* Primal Blueprint Publishing, 2013.

Denise Minger is a brilliant self-taught data junkie and in this book lays bare food politics in America and what is healthy nutrition. She dissects each of the recommended diets in America from the four food groups through the pyramids. She also reanalyzed the data from Colin

Campbell's *The China Study* showing that, among other things, fish from wild sources also was associated with lower cancer rates.

Scott Jurek. *Eat & Run: My Unlikely Journey to Ultramarathon Greatness.* (2012). Houghton Mifflin Harcourt Publishing.

Scott Jurek is the first male star performer of ultramarathons. He is also a vegan. This book is his life story from his childhood near Duluth Minnesota to setting new records in the Western States 100-mile Endurance Run winning it six years in a row. His journey of being lean and fit is inspiring and he continues to break limits just setting a new record for completing the Appalachian Trail in 47 days.

Dan Buetner. *The Blue Zones Solution: Eating and Living Like the World's Healthiest People* (2015). National Geographic Society.

Who can argue about the ingredients of the healthiest people on Earth? What I find fascinating about the nutrition of the Blue Zone populations is that they are mostly very healthy and the people are lean and fit and relaxed. Most do eat some of the toxic carbohydrates such as breads. They live an average of eight years longer than other populations. I wonder how long they would live with optimal nutrition without the inflammatory foods?

Websites:

curealiy.com Hosted by William Davis, MD

Drperlmutter.com Hosted by David Perlmutter, MD

Drhyman.com Hosted by Mark Hyman, MD

rawfoodsos.com Hosted by Denise Minger

Appendix III

Other Nutrition Articles

Spice is Nice

Internal Medicine Alert
September 15, 2015;37(17):129-130

Synopsis: The habitual consumption of spicy foods is associated with reduced mortality independent of other risk factors for death.

Source: Lv J, Qi L, Yu C, et al. Consumption of spicy foods and total and cause specific mortality: population based cohort study. BMJ. 2015;351:h3942.

A group of Chinese investigators conducted a prospective cohort study between 2004 and 2008 and followed 512,891 adults aged 30-79 until the end of 2013. Participants completed a questionnaire and were divided into four groups based on their reported intake of spices: never, 1-2 days/week, 3-5 days/week and 6-7 days/week. The spices identified were fresh chili pepper, dried chili pepper, chili sauce, chili oil and other spices. Ten survey sites were resurveyed in 2008 to confirm the continued intake of spices. Other risk factors for death such as socioeconomic status, life style behaviors, nutritional intake, presence of chronic conditions, body mass index, fasting blood glucose and blood pressure were also measured.

Local health insurance databases were used to determine death and its causes. Seven categories of death were used: cancer, ischemic heart disease, cerebrovascular disease, diabetes mellitus, respiratory disease, infections and other causes.

The results show that participants who ate spicy foods 6 or 7 days a week showed a 14% relative risk reduction in total mortality compared with those who ate spicy foods less than once a week. Any regular consumption of spices reduced mortality. The reduction was seen in deaths from cancer, ischemic heart disease and respiratory disease. No associations were significant in the other causes of death. Men and women showed a similar risk reduction.

Commentary

Spices have a long history in the culinary world and the spice trade is part of the history of civilization. There is a worldwide trend of increased use of spices as flavorings in foods[1,2]. In China, chili pepper is among the most popular spicy foods consumed.

Beneficial effects of spices have been studied, and their bioactive ingredients such as capsaicin have been shown to reduce cancer[2-4]. Red pepper has been found to decrease appetite and reduce the rate of overweight and obesity[5]. Spices exhibit antibacterial activity and have an impact on the gut microbiota populations in a way that may reduce the risk of diabetes, cardiovascular disease, liver cirrhosis and cancer [6-8].

This study reinforces the emerging science that suggests our nutrition should focus on the wisdom of the ages more than depend on recent processed foods. Spices have a place among the healthy ingredients of a cuisine. Like with coffee and tea, it is nice when culinary pleasure combines with better health.

References

1. Tapsell LC, Hemphill I, Cobiac L, et al. Health benefits of herbs and spices: the past, the present, the future. Med J Aust. 2006;185(4 Suppl):S4-24.
2. Kaefer CM, Milner JA. The role of herbs and spices in cancer prevention. J Nutr Biochem. 2008;19:347-361.
3. Billing J, Sherman PW. Antimicrobial functions of spices: why some like it hot. Q Rev Biol. 198;73:3-49.
4. Aggarwal BB, Van Kuiken ME, Iyer LH, et al. Molecular targets of nutriceuticals derived from dietary spices: potential role in suppression of inflammation and tumorigenesis. Exp Biol Med. 2009;234:825-849.
5. Yoshioka M, St-Pierre S, Drapeau V, et al. Effects of red pepper and caffeine consumption on 24 hour energy balance in subjects given free access to foods. Br J Nutr. 2001;85:203-211.
6. Tang WHW, Wang ZE, Levison BS, et al. Intestinal microbial metabolism of phosphatidylcholine and cardiovascular risk. N Engl J Med. 2013;368:1575-1584.
7. Qin N, Yang F, Li A, et al. Alterations of the human gut microbiome in liver cirrhosis. Nature. 2014;513:59-64.
8. Qin J, Li Y, Cai Z, et al. A metagenome-wide association study of gut microbiota in type 2 diabetes. Nature. 2012;490:55-60.

Nutrition Therapy for Hypertension Using the Nitric Oxide Pathway

Internal Medicine Alert
October 5, 2015;37(19):146-147

Synopsis: Daily one-time ingestion of inorganic nitrate from beet juice consistently lowered blood pressure in hypertensive patients by an amount comparable to single drug therapy.

Source: Kapil V, Khambata RS, Robertson A, et al. Dietary Nitrate Provides Sustained Blood Pressure Lowering Hypertensive Patients. *Hypertension.* 2015;65:320-327.

This carefully controlled randomized trial was performed in London comparing the use of inorganic nitrate found in beet juice and placebo in controlling blood pressure in hypertensive patients. 64 patients underwent a 4-week trial of drinking one 250 ml bottle of beet juice daily and 4 weeks of a placebo beet juice with the nitrate removed. There was a two-week washout period. The sequence of juice ingestion was randomized into two groups. All patients were mildly hypertensive and had no renal impairment. Those on medication continued their therapy during the trial. Adults were studied from age 18 to 85 years.

Blood pressure was measured in three ways for each patient: one-daily home blood pressure, a 24-hour ambulatory blood pressure measurement near the end of the 4-week period, and clinic blood pressure measurements. All patients ingesting the nitrate containing beet juice had reductions in blood pressure and those on placebo did not. The blood pressure reductions were similar for all three methods. Home blood pressure was reduced by 8.1 mmHg (3.8-12.4) systolic and 3.8 mmHg (0.7-6.9) diastolic. Clinic blood pressures were reduced by 7.7 mmHg (3.6-11) and 2.4 mmHg (0.0-4.9) diastolic. Ambulatory blood pressures were reduced by 7.7 mmHg (3.5-11.8) systolic and 5.2 mmHg (2.7-7.7) diastolic. These reductions were sustained over the 4 weeks.

In addition, the beet juice was associated with improvements in vascular function through vasodilatation and improved endothelial function. There were no adverse side effects of ingesting the beet juice except for the change in color of the urine and feces.

It is well known that nitric oxide (NO) in the blood is a potent vasodilator. The mechanism of action of the dietary inorganic nitrate being converted to NO has only recently been understood[1,2]. Inorganic nitrate is absorbed in the small intestine and is extracted from the blood via the salivary glands of the mouth[3]. The microbiome in the mouth converts the nitrate to nitrite[1,2]. So much for the GI tract being a one way street! Swallowing the saliva the nitrite enters the circulation where it meets enzymes, nitrite reductases that convert it to NO in the circulation[4]. The NO then causes vasodilation and blood pressure lowering. This is a uniquely physiologic phenomenon that has defied attempts at pharmacotherapy. Organic nitrites such as nitroglycerin suffer from problems of endothelial dysfunction and tachyphylaxis[5].

Commentary

This study is the first to show durable blood pressure reduction from the nutritional intake of nitrates. It is an example of how nutrition has the potential to treat the most common of chronic diseases, hypertension.

The study indicates the use of beetroot juice. What the English call beetroot is simply beets or red beets in North America. Besides beets, vegetables high in nitrates include spinach, celery, rugola and other lettuce, cress and chervil. The evidence would suggest that a daily consumption of a healthy portion of these vegetables may reduce the incidence of hypertension, and help treat it when it exists. Juicing vegetables would be a convenient way to ensure a consistent amount of nitrates in the daily diet.

The 12th century physician, Maimonides, stated that "No disease that can be treated with diet should be treated with any other means[6]." Nutrition as therapy is underdeveloped in Western medicine. In China and other Eastern countries the medical pharmacy is loaded with nutritional herbs and the hospital may have a vegetable garden on the premises. Western physicians may look at this practice as quaint and not evidence based through controlled trials.

Kapil and his colleagues are to be commended for this carefully controlled trial as to how a vegetable product used daily significantly reduces blood pressure in hypertensive patients. The role of the microbiome in this mechanism is most interesting and suggests there are many more complex nutritional therapies yet to be understood and discovered.

References

1. Larsen FJ, Ekblom B, Sahlin K, et al. Effects of dietary nitrate on blood pressure in healthy volunteers. N Engl J Med. 2006;355:2792-2793.
2. Webb AJ, Patel N, Loukogeorgakis S, et al. Acute blood pressure lowering, vasoprotective, and antiplatelet properties of dietary nitrate via bioconversion to nitratet. Hypertension. 2008;51:784-790.
3. Tannenbaum SR, Weisman M, Fett D. The effect of nitrate intake on nitrite formation in human saliva. Food Cosmet Toxicol. 1976;14:549-552.
4. Cosby K, Partovi KS, Crawford JH, et al. Nitrite reduction to nitric oxide by deoxyhemoglobin vasodilates the human circulation. Nat Med. 2003;9:1498-1505.
5. Gori T, Mak SS, Kelly S, Parker JD. Evidence supporting abnormalities in nitric oxide synthase function induced by nitroglycerin in humans. J Am Coll Cardiol. 2001;38:1096-1101.
6. Wikiquote: Maimodides. En.m.wikiquote.org

The Mediterranean Diet Plus Extra Virgin Olive Oil May Improve or Maintain Cognitive Function in Mature Adults. Low Fat Diet May Result in Cognitive Decline.

Internal Medicine Alert
Accepted, publication pending

Synopsis: A controlled trial of adults age 55 to 80 showed that intake of a Mediterranean Diet plus 1 liter of Extra Virgin Olive Oil each week improved or maintained cognitive function compared with controls on a low fat diet who showed cognitive decline.

Source: Valls-Pedret C, Sala-Vila A, Serra-Mir M, et al. Mediterranean Diet and Age-Related Cognitive Decline: A Randomized Clinical Trial. JAMA Intern Med. 2015;175:1094-1103.

This is a post-hoc analysis of a study in Barcelona, Spain looking at antioxidant supplementation in a population of men aged 55-80 and women aged 60-80 followed between 2003 and 2009. 447 cognitively healthy volunteers, roughly half men and women, were randomly assigned to three groups: a Mediterranean diet plus one liter of extra virgin olive oil/week, a Mediterranean diet plus 30g/wk of mixed nuts (walnuts, hazelnuts and almonds), and a low fat diet as the control group. All of the volunteers were at high risk for cardiovascular disease with 55% having type 2 diabetes and the rest having at least 3 of the following 4 risk factors: hypertension, dyslipidemia, overweight/obesity, and a family history of early onset coronary heart disease. None had active cardiovascular disease at the time of the trial.

An experienced neuropsychologist performed a battery of cognitive tests at the beginning of the study and again about 4 years later. The drop-out rate was similar for all three groups and 340 volunteers (76%) completed the two cognitive screenings.

The 127 volunteers who were on the Mediterranean diet plus extra virgin olive oil showed slight improvement in the cognitive tests, the 112 volunteers on the Mediterranean diet plus nuts showed no significant change, and the 97 on a low fat diet showed some decline in their cognitive tests.

The authors conclude that in an older population, a Mediterranean diet supplemented with olive oil or nuts is associated with improved cognitive function compared with controls on a low fat diet.

Commentary

This study is small and inconclusive but does suggest two important things. First eating healthy may preserve cognitive function. The authors do not spell out what is meant by the Mediterranean diet but we must assume it is rich in healthy vegetables, fruit and seafood. Not clear is the role of pasta. The amount of olive oil consumed in the one group may not be practical, and it is not clear how much olive oil and nuts were part of Mediterranean diet in both groups.

The second suggestion is that low fat consumption may be associated with cognitive decline. David Perlmutter in his well-referenced books *Grain Brain*[1] and *Brain Maker*[2] underscores the importance of healthy fats in brain health. Our brain is made up of lots of cholesterol so encourage people to eat the yolks.

Much more work needs to be done to clarify the role of diet and cognitive function. The gut-brain axis is being scientifically illuminated in a way that medicine will need to start taking nutrition much more seriously[2,3]. What is clear is that the low-fat diet recommendations of the 70s, 80s and 90s are obsolete. The Mediterranean diet appears to be one of the best candidates for a nutrition recommendation.

References

1. Perlmutter D, Grain Brain. New York; Little Brown, 2013.
2. Perlmutter D. Brain Maker. New York: Little, Brown and Co. 2015.
3. Petra AI, Panagiotidou S, Hatziagelaki E, et al. Gut-Microbiota-Brain Axis and its Effect on Neuropsychiatric Disorders With Suspected Immune Dysfunction. Clin Ther. 2015;37:984-995.

Eat Right, Preserve Your Memory and Stay Happy!

Internal Medicine Alert
Accepted, publication pending

Synopsis: Greater intake of unhealthy food and lower intake of nutrient dense food is associated with a smaller hippocampus over four years in adults aged 60-64.

Source: Jacka FN, Cherbuin N, Ansley KJ, et al. Western diet is associated with a smaller hippocampus: a longitudinal investigation. BMC Medicine. 2015;13:215-222.

A team of investigators from Australia used a database of 2551 adults living in and around Canberra who participated in the Personality and Total Health (PATH) Through Life Project starting in 2001. A subgroup of 255 persons were in the age 60-64 cohort and had both a diet survey and an MRI initially and four years later. Diets were self-reported and put on a scale from "prudent" (healthy) emphasizing fresh vegetables, salad, fruit and grilled fish to "Western" (unhealthy) emphasizing roast meat, sausages, hamburgers, steak, chips and soft drinks.

Significant differences were found with diet and change in the size of the hippocampus on MRI. Every one standard deviation increase in the healthy dietary pattern was associated with a 45.7 mm larger left hippocampal volume, while a higher consumption of the unhealthy foods was independently associated with a 52.6 mm smaller left hippocampal volume. These relationships were independent of variables such as age, gender, education, work status, depressive symptoms, medication, physical activity, smoking, hypertension and diabetes.

This is the first study that demonstrated a relationship between and diet and the size of the hippocampus in humans. Such an association has been shown in animals[1,2]. The authors propose a variety of mechanisms for this change, such as inflammation, oxidative stress, and the gut microbiome.

Commentary

The hippocampus is a part of the brain associated with learning, memory and mood regulation. The hippocampus has been specifically implicated as a site for depression[3]. Environmental factors, especially nutrition and physical activity, have been shown to reduce or increase through neurogenesis the size of the hippocampus[4]. This study shows that just four years in the sixth decade makes a significant difference in the size of the hippocampus depending on diet.

I recently read an amazing book, *The Story of the Human Body*, by the Harvard evolutionary biologist Daniel Lieberman[5]. Lieberman traces the development of humans from the chimpanzee through the hominoids to our long hunter-gatherer period. He then describes the impact of the agrarian and industrial ages on our bodies and our health. The impact has been mostly negative. Sure we are living longer than ever (for now) but we have a multitude of diseases not known to the animal kingdom. Most importantly we have a growing epidemic of cognitive impairment and dementia.

Nutrition may have a preeminent role in the health of our brains. The emergence of understanding the gut microbiome in brain health has been presented in IMA recently[6]. Inflammation appears to be the common denominator in most chronic diseases involving the body and mind. Unhealthy foods induce inflammation in the body, something that deserves much more attention in our social policies, public health and medical practice.

References

1. Heyward FD, Walton RG, Carle MS, et al. Adult mice maintained on a high-fat diet exhibit object location memory deficits and reduced hippocampal SIRT 1 gene expression. Neurobiol Learn Mem. 2012;98:25-32.

2. Morrison CD, Pistell PJ, Ingram DK, et al. High fat diet increases hippocampal oxidative stress and cognitive impairment in aged mice: Implications for decreased Nrf2 signaling. J Neurochem. 2010;114:1581-1589.

3. Sapolsky RM. Glucocorticoids and hippocampal atrophy in neuropsychiatric disorders. Arch Gen Psychiatry. 2000;57:925-935.

4. Das S, Basu A. Inflammation: A new candidate in modulating adult neurogenesis: J Neurosci Res. 2008;86:1199-1208.

5. Lieberman DE. The Story of the Human Body: Evolution, Health and Disease. New York: Pantheon Books, 2013.

6. Scherger JE. You Are What You Feed Your Gut Microbiome. Internal Medicine Alert. August 29, 2015;37(16):121-122.

JOSEPH E. SCHERGER, MD, MPH

ABOUT THE AUTHOR

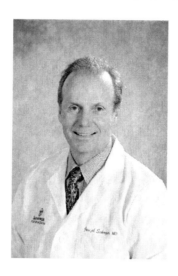

Joseph E. Scherger, M.D., M.P.H., is Vice President for Primary Care and Marie E. Pinizzotto, MD, Chair of Academic Affairs at Eisenhower Medical Center in Rancho Mirage, California. Dr. Scherger is Clinical Professor of Family Medicine at the Keck School of Medicine at the University of Southern California (USC). Dr. Scherger is a leader in transforming office practice and has special interests in nutrition and wellness. He is the author of *40 Years in Family Medicine* self-published with Amazon in 2014.

Originally from Delphos, Ohio, Dr. Scherger graduated from the University of Dayton in 1971, summa cum laude. He graduated from the UCLA School of Medicine in 1975, and was elected to Alpha Omega Alpha. He completed a Family Medicine Residency and a Masters in Public Health at the University of Washington in 1978. From 1978-80, he served in the National Health Service Corps in Dixon, California, as a migrant health physician. From 1981-92, Dr. Scherger divided his time between private practice in Dixon and teaching medical students and residents at UC Davis. From 1988-91, he was a Fellow in the Kellogg National Fellowship Program, focusing on health care reform and quality of life. From 1992-1996, he was Vice President for Family Practice and Primary Care Education at Sharp HealthCare in San Diego. From 1996-2001, he was the Chair of the Department of Family Medicine and the Associate Dean for Primary Care at the University of California Irvine. From 2001-2003, Dr. Scherger served as founding dean of the Florida State University College of Medicine.

Dr. Scherger has received numerous awards, including being recognized as a "Top Doc" in San Diego for 6 consecutive years, 2004-2009. He was voted Outstanding Clinical Instructor at the University of California, Davis School of Medicine in 1984, 1989 and 1990. In 1989, he was Family Physician of the Year by the American Academy of Family Physicians and the California Academy of Family Physicians. In 1986, he was President of the Society of Teachers of Family Medicine. In 1992, Dr. Scherger was elected to the Institute of Medicine of the National Academy of Sciences. In 1994, he received the Thomas W. Johnson Award for Family Practice Education from the American Academy of Family Physicians. In 2000, he was selected by the UC Irvine medical students for the AAMC Humanism in Medicine Award. He received the Lynn and Joan Carmichael Recognition Award from the Society of Teachers of Family Medicine in 2012. He served on the Institute of Medicine Committee on the Quality of Health Care in America from 1998-2001. Dr. Scherger served on the Board of Directors of the American Academy of Family Physicians and the American Board of Family Medicine. From 2005-2010 he served as Consulting

Medical Director for Quality and Informatics at Lumetra Healthcare Solutions.

Dr. Scherger serves on the editorial board of *Medical Economics* and is an Assistant Editor of *Family Medicine*. He is a Senior Fellow with the Estes Park Institute on Information Technology and Quality Improvement. He was the Men's Health expert and a consultant for Revolution Health, 2006-09, and he has covered California for eDocAmerica since 2003. He was Editor-in-Chief of *Hippocrates*, published by the Massachusetts Medical Society, from 1999-2001. He was the first Medical Editor of *Family Practice Management*. He has authored more than 400 medical publications and has given over 1000 invited presentations.

Dr. Scherger enjoys an active family life with his wife, Carol, and two sons, Adrian and Gabriel. He has completed 37 marathons, nine 50K and five 50 mile ultramarathon trail runs.

CPSIA information can be obtained
at www.ICGtesting.com
Printed in the USA
LVOW12s1632110716

495870LV00024B/1454/P